MW01100556

PHACOEMULSIFICATION

New Technology and Clinical Application

PHACOEMULSIFICATION

New Technology and Clinical Application

I. Howard Fine, MD

Oregon Eye Associates
Eugene, Oregon

SLACK Incorporated, 6900 Grove Road, Thorofare, NJ 08086-9447

Publisher: John H. Bond
Acquisitions Editor: Amy E. Drummond
Associate Editor: Jennifer J. Cahill
Art Director: Linda Baker

Phacoemulsification: new technology and clinical application/[edited] by I. Howard Fine.
p. cm.
Includes bibliographical references and index.
ISBN 1-55642-273-3
1. Phacoemulsification. 2. Phacoemulsification—Equipment and supplies. I. Fine, I. Howard.
[DNLM: 1. Cataract Extraction—methods. 2. Cataract Extraction—instrumentation. WW 260 P5319 1995]
RE451.P47 1995
617.7′42059—dc20
DNLM/DLC
for Library of Congress 95-37025

Printed in the United States of America

Published by: SLACK Incorporated
6900 Grove Road
Thorofare, NJ 08086-9447 USA
Telephone: 609-848-1000
Fax: 609-853-5991

Contact SLACK Incorporated for more information about other books in this field or about the availability of our books from distributors outside the United States.

Last digit is print number: 10 9 8 7 6 5 4 3 2 1

Dedication

This book is dedicated to Ephraim Friedman, MD, who taught me that elegance and excellence in eye surgery occur only when there is commitment; to Simmons Lessell, MD, who taught me that initiating change in surgical technique requires courage; and to Howard M. Leibowitz, MD, who trained me and championed me as well.

Contents

Contents

Acknowledgments

All phaco surgeons owe a debt of gratitude to the manufacturers of phacoemulsification equipment whose commitment to improving cataract surgery has made such a difference in the lives of so many patients. I appreciate the fact that they have allowed me to work with their equipment and come to understand it. The operating room staff of the Oregon Eye Surgery Center, through flexibility and insight, have facilitated the introduction of new technology to my own operating room. Their understanding of the equipment and underlying principles has helped me improve my surgical technique. I continue to be awed by Mary Ellen Watson, COMT, my surgical assistant and research associate. She lives through learning curves with grace and composure, never losing sight of the task or the goal. My editors at SLACK Incorporated, Amy Drummond and Jennifer Cahill, have always given me good advice with just the right touch. Finally, I want to thank my wife, Vicky, the ultimate editor in my life. She creates prose and figures of speech out of linguistic turmoil, often late at night and on an empty stomach.

Contributing Authors

Aziz Anis, MD
Lincoln, Nebraska

D. Michael Colvard, MD
Encino, California

Jack M. Dodick, MD
New York, New York

Daniel M. Eichenbaum, MD
Murphy, North Carolina

I. Howard Fine, MD
Eugene, Oregon

Harry B. Grabow, MD
Sarasota, Florida

John D. Hunkeler, MD
Kansas City, Missouri

Charles D. Kelman, MD
New York, New York

Richard P. Kratz, MD
Newport Beach, California

Richard J. Mackool, MD
New York, New York

Samuel Masket, MD
West Hills, California

Laurence T. D. Sperber, MD
New York, New York

Roger F. Steinert, MD
Boston, Massachusetts

Richard Thorlakson, MD
Bellevue, Washington

For 20 years after the introduction of phacoemulsification, machine parameters were set arbitrarily by the manufacturer. I say arbitrarily because I could rarely discern any rational thought behind the factory-recommended vacuum and flow rate settings. Teaching and learning phaco in those early days were, in some ways, easier tasks than they are today. If one used the same machine with manufacturer-set parameters, the beginner only needed to mimic the intraocular maneuvers of the teacher in order to obtain similar effects.

In the late 1980s, some surgeons (among them my friends Robert Osher, MD, of Cincinnati, Ohio and Robert Schnipper, MD, of Jacksonville, Fla) began to alter the parameters of flow and vacuum, resulting in improved techniques and outcomes. In the early 1990s, we saw the introduction of dramatic new technology in phacoemulsification with expanded choices in parameter settings, multiple programmable features, microprocessor controls, and new designs and technology impacting all of the components of the system from the phacoemulsification tip at the handpiece to ultrasonic generators, tubing, cassettes, consoles, right down to the foot pedal. Now, to mimic another's technique, we must know all about his or her parameters in order to achieve similar results.

That is only part of the story of the new phacoemulsification technology. Today we have options and capabilities never previously available, but to take advantage of them we must understand how the equipment works. This is a new requirement because in the past it wasn't necessary to understand the machinery. We can rise above past and present limitations in technique only by understanding the technology, using it, and expanding it. This book was conceived with that thought in mind.

The authors of this book are all superb technicians and dedicated teachers. Each chapter discusses the technology from a clinical perspective. It then explains how that technology is applied and how that technology has impacted the author's personal phacoemulsification technique.

When I was a college undergraduate, most students had radios in their rooms. A few of my classmates had high fidelity sets, which were relatively new at the time. Some of these hi-fi sets, however, sounded no better than my little radio; their owners didn't understand how to use any of the options other than the on/off switch and the volume control. Other sets sounded incredible; full use of the technology had achieved the sensation that an entire symphony orchestra was present in a small room. And so it is with "high fidelity" phacoemulsification.

I. Howard Fine, MD
Oregon Eye Associates
Eugene, Oregon

Chapter 1

HISTORY OF PHACOEMULSIFICATION

Charles D. Kelman, MD

A resident in ophthalmology today, seeing his or her first cataract operation performed by a surgeon who uses Kelman phacoemulsification, might wonder how it could be performed any other way. Seated comfortably at the operating microscope, the surgeon makes a tiny incision, neatly peels open the anterior capsule, emulsifies and aspirates the lens within the remaining capsule, and then, through the same incision, inserts a foldable lens. On the first postoperative day, in most cases, it is difficult to tell with the naked eye which eye has been operated.

In contrast, in 1960, when I finished my residency at Wills Eye Hospital, general anesthesia was common, no microscopes were used for any ophthalmic surgery anywhere in the world (except for Richard Perritt, MD, a surgeon in Chicago), a 180° incision was made, a large sector iridectomy was performed, and then the lens was grasped by a capsule forceps and the entire lens was pulled from the eye. Eight or more sutures closed the incision, and the patient remained hospitalized for 7 to 10 days. The eyes were red, the lids swollen and irritated for up to 6 weeks.

One might ask how the idea for phaco came to me. Did I one day think "I'll just take an ultrasonic needle and remove the cataract that way"? As brilliant as that leap of thought would have been, I cannot pretend to claim credit for making it. Actually, it is so far from the truth that the real answer serves to illustrate a point: the final solution to a problem is usually far afield from the first attempts at its solution.

First, the impetus for wanting to find a better way to remove cataracts. I was in the process of writing a grant application to the John A. Hartford Foundation to investigate the effects of freezing on the eye, and after finishing the final draft, I went to bed. But I couldn't sleep. The application seemed boring; I knew that the foundation looked to support breakthrough procedures, not boring scientific studies. I knew in my heart that the application would be rejected. I needed something exciting but I didn't know what. Without knowing what I was doing, I put my subconscious mind to work, and went to bed.

Sometime in the night I got out of bed and wrote a phrase that would forever change my life, and would forever change the practice of cataract surgery. That phrase was: "The author will also find a way to remove a cataract through a tiny incision, eliminating the need for hospitalization, general anesthesia, and dramatically shortening the recovery period." That statement looked well on paper. I had no idea how I would accomplish this feat. I was, however, confident that I could do so easily. This confidence sprang from three factors:

- I had quite easily discovered cryoretinopexy, and had published the first paper on that subject.[1]
- I had quite easily co-discovered (Krwawicz, in Poland, had also independently discovered the same thing) cryoextraction of cataracts.[2]
- I was blissfully and naively unaware of the complexity of the task I had set out for myself.

It is certainly possible that had I known the number of problems I would have to solve, I would have been intimidated and might have never started. It is for this reason that often people outside of a particular discipline are able to make breakthroughs. Those more knowledgeable are too aware of the difficulties.

The Hartford Foundation director, E. Pierre Roy, called me a few days later to tell me that he was not interested in the effects of freezing on the eye, but that he would give the grant for the new cataract operation. I was ecstatic! This was going to be easy.

The first "method" for removing the lens through a small incision revolved around a collapsible "butterfly net" (Figure 1-1), the net portion being made out of condom-thin latex. The idea I had was to dilate the pupil, instill an enzyme to loosen the zonule, turn the patient over on his or her face and vibrate his or her head with a manual vibrator until the lens fell into the anterior chamber, then instill acetylcholine to constrict the pupil. Once the cataract was trapped in the anterior chamber, the collapsed latex net would be introduced to trap the cataract, which would then be simply mushed up with a needle until the net and the squashed cataract could be pulled through the small incision. It is important for the reader to note how far from the sophisticated phaco machines this original, naive idea was. It would have been so easy to listen to those who said to me, "I told you you couldn't do it," and admit defeat, just as it may be easy for you the reader to abandon your first idea on a subject and never get to the second generation, the third, the fourth, the fifth, the sixth, until you come up with a solution totally unrelated to your original idea.

This "cat in the bag method" could not be made to work. (All attempts with this device were made on animal and eye bank eyes.) It was too traumatic to the cornea, the bag was too thick, the bag took too much volume in the anterior chamber, and the bag kept breaking. It had taken 6 months to fabricate this "butterfly net" and to test it. I had used up one sixth of my 3-year grant, and I began to worry. I then began investigating devices that would break up a cataract, so that it could be irrigated and aspirated from the eye.

Various drills, rotary devices, and various types of microblenders were constructed and tried (Figures 1-2 through 1-4). Each failed for several reasons. If the iris was touched with a rotating tip, it would immediately

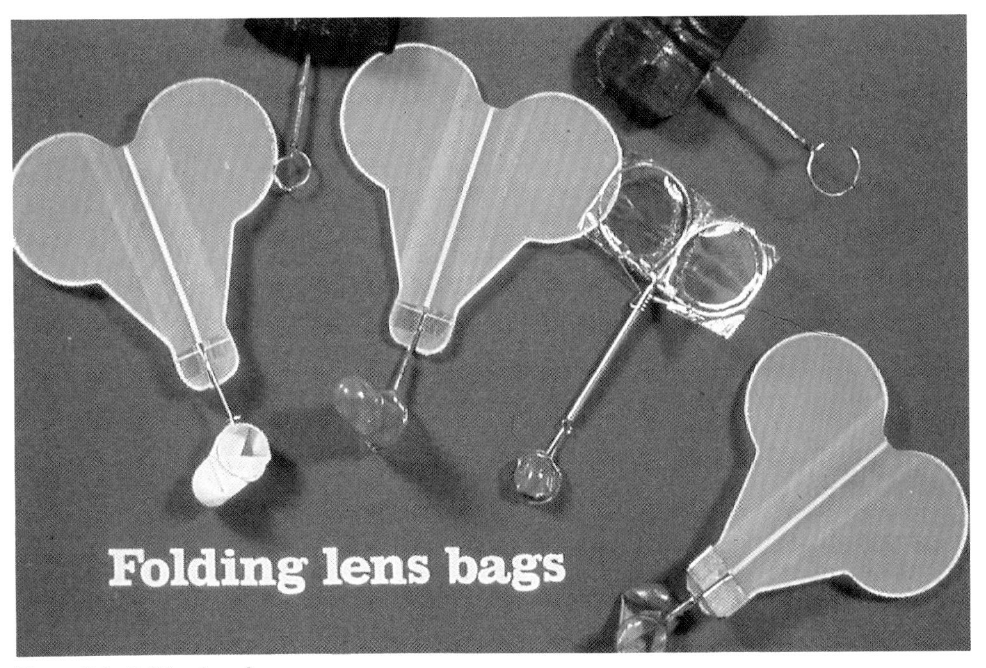

Figure 1-1. Folding lens bags.

become completely ensnared and a total 360° iridodialysis would inadvertently be performed. Usually, uncontrollable hemorrhage would ensue. Furthermore, the iris did not even have to be close to the rotating tip. The eddy currents set up within the chamber were enough to draw the iris to the rotating tip and instantaneously disinsert and remove it.

The second obstacle to fast rotating devices was that the eddy currents set up in the anterior chamber would throw lens particles against the endothelium and completely denude it in a few seconds, leading to permanent opacification and vascularization. Thirdly, the lens itself when caught on the rotating tip would also spin in the chamber with the consequent destruction of the endothelium. The microblender (Figure 1-5) with needless rotating in opposite directions was intended to prevent the lens from spinning, but it was unsatisfactory. It also increased the chances of incarcerating the iris in the two rotating tips. Slow turning drills (Figure 1-6) were designed, but these, too, were unable to prevent the lens from turning. Rocking vibrators still rubbed off endothelium. These abandoned devices are similar to the rotorooter-type devices which others are re-evaluating at present. Steps were taken to fix the lens from the opposite side with the use of the prongs. The sharp tips, however, endangered the posterior capsule. Low frequency vibrators were tried, but the lens merely vibrated with the tip. None of the aforementioned devices were ever used clinically, as they were considered dangerous and ineffective.

Two years, and most of the grant money, had now elapsed. The solution of this problem had become more than a challenge—it had become an obsession.

In analyzing the difficulties I had had so far, it became clear that the main problem was that the lens was moving, rotating, or vibrating inside of the anterior chamber and, therefore, rubbing against the endothelium. This realization eventually led to the solution only a few months before the expiration of the grant. At this time, it became obvious that in order for the lens to remain stationary in the chamber, the acceleration of the moving tip against it had to be high enough so that the standing inertia of the lens would not be overcome; in other words, high enough acceleration was required so that the lens could not back away, vibrate, or rotate with the tip. To demonstrate this principle, imagine a sharp knife slowly pushing against a punching bag. The punching bag will move with the knife. If, however, the knife is quickly plunged against the bag, the knife will enter and the bag will not move. In this analogy, the punching bag represents the lens and the knife represents the tool used to enter the lens. This high acceleration could

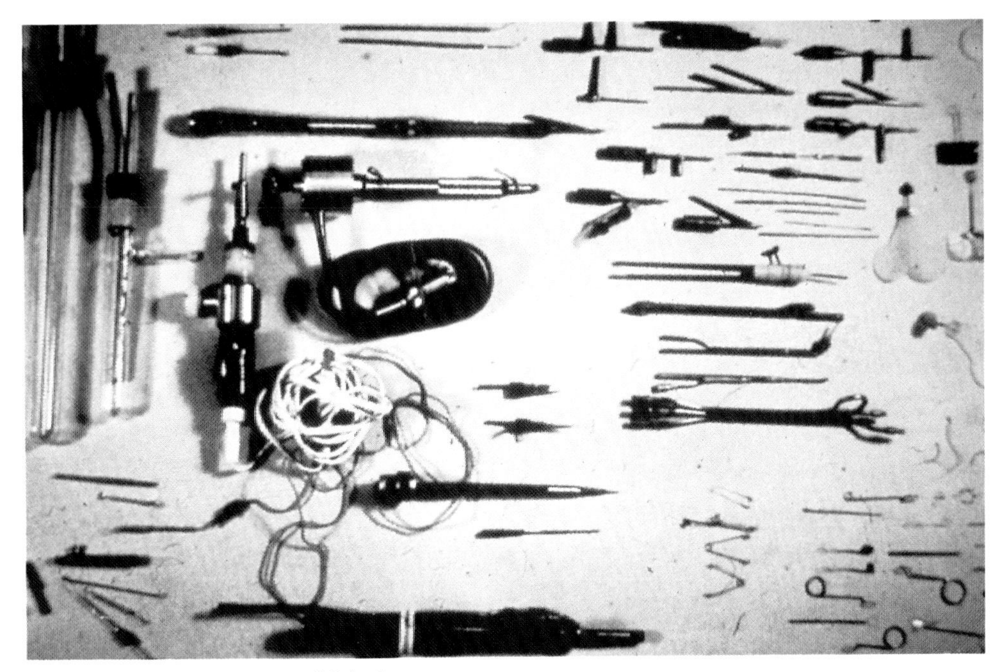

Figure 1-2. Various unsuccessful devices.

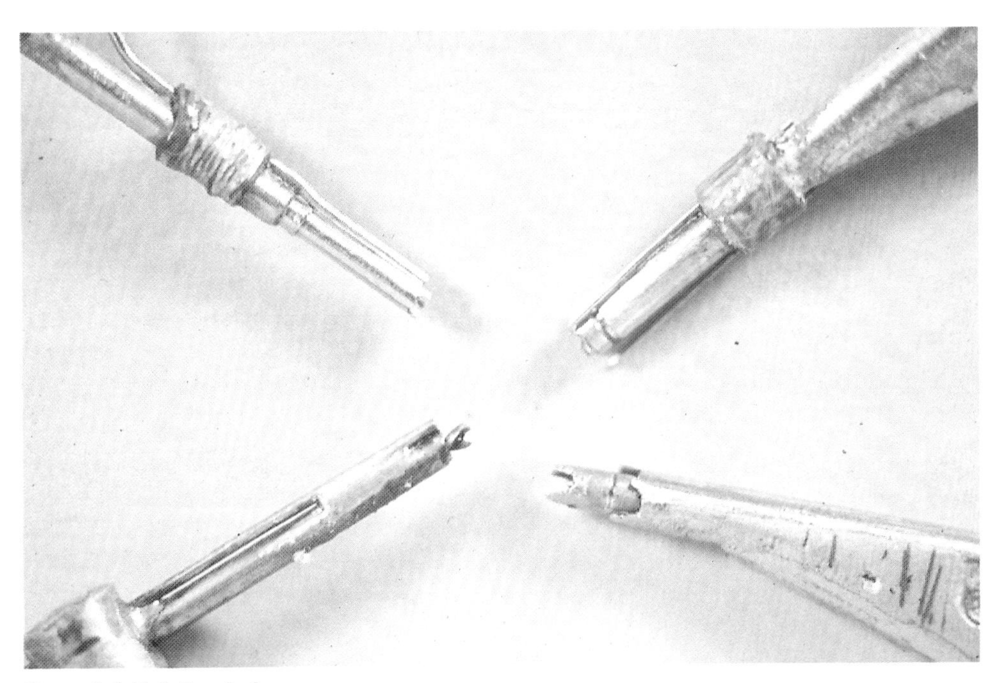

Figure 1-3. Rotating devices.

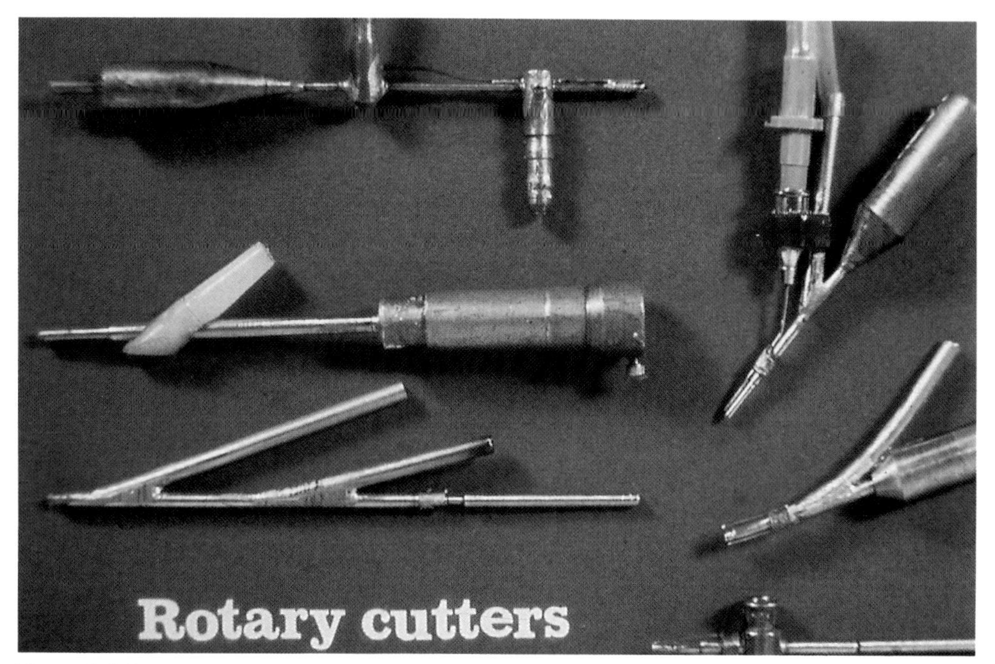

Figure 1-4. Rotary cutters.

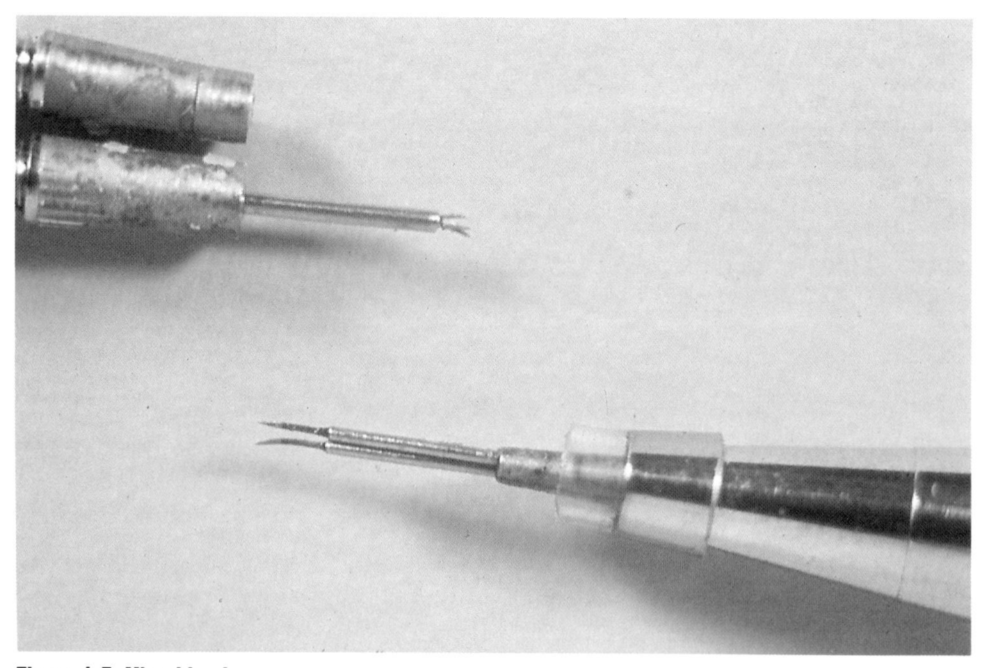

Figure 1-5. Microblenders.

only be achieved with an ultrasonic frequency. Early experiments with a dental ultrasonic unit using irrigation only and a nonlongitudinal motion were encouraging, but were clinically unsuccessful because of the high energy radiated and the relative inefficiency requiring many minutes of ultrasonic time in the anterior chamber. Substitution of a longitudinal motion at the tip was introduced to prevent disinsertion of the iris and to reduce radiation. This type of motion also significantly reduced flaking. (Originally published in 1974. Published courtesy of the American Academy of Ophthalmology.)[3]

Once I had discovered the method of breaking up the lens, I thought the rest would be easy. It wasn't. There were three types of problems lurking ahead which, as they were discovered, had to be overcome:

- Surgical problems
- Instrument problems
- Political problems

Surgical Problems

Pupil Constriction

In the first attempts to do phacoemulsification, the pupil constricted during the surgery. There had to be new drugs and methods to maintain dilation.

In the early cases, the pupil constricted rapidly in the procedure, since we did not have potent mydriatics at the time. At first, I performed large sector iridectomies so that I could see behind the iris, but in many cases the iris became aspirated into the tip and became badly frayed. Because of this problem, I began to bring the lens into the anterior chamber before performing the phaco and before the pupil constricted. For several years I then taught anterior chamber phaco, which I believe is still a viable alternative to posterior chamber phaco, for those less skilled. There is a slight increase in endothelial cell loss over posterior chamber phaco, but not enough to be significant.

After a few years, mydriatics were placed in the irrigating solution and anti-inflammatory drops were used on the cornea in combination with more powerful mydriatics. Once viscoelastics came into use, they too aided in pupillary dilation, and posterior chamber phaco became much easier. For those pupils that are fibrotic, several models of iris hooks are available.

Anterior Capsular Opening

A method of opening the anterior capsule had to be developed which would be consistent, exposing the lens, but not extending to the zonules.

My first attempts to incise the anterior capsule in several directions with criss-crossing lines taught me that these incisions in the capsule, if subjected to traction, could extend around the anterior surface of the lens into the zonule, and perhaps even onto the posterior capsule. One day, I observed on an animal eye that if I used a dull cystotome rather than a sharp one, instead of cutting the capsule, the cystotome tore it. And that tear was always in the form of a triangle. I named this technique the Christmas Tree Opening (Figure 1-7). If I could rewrite history, I would call it a triangular capsulorhexis, a more accurate description, and one that would place it in its proper historical position, the forerunner of the continuous tear capsulorhexis. Once the triangular tear was made, the pie-shaped flap would be grasped with a forceps, gently extracted, and then cut at its base. This method was in general use until the "can opener technique" was introduced, and then finally the continuous tear technique widely used today.

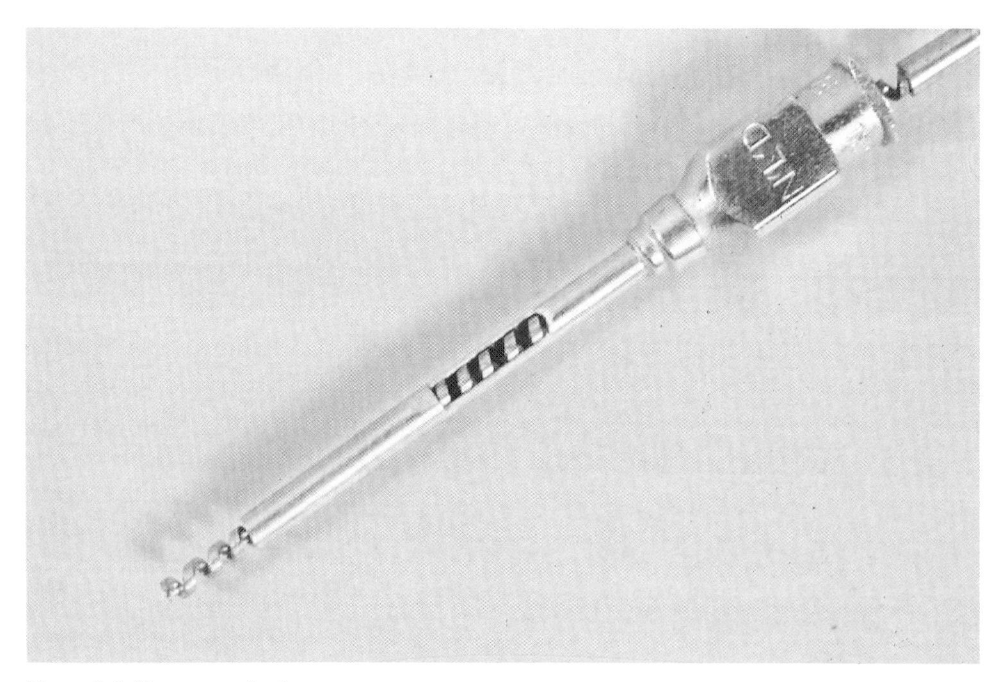

Figure 1-6. Worm gear feeder.

Magnification and Visualization

Using loupes (the standard method of magnification at the time), the magnification was not adequate. Using existing surgical microscopes gave no depth perception, since the lighting was flat, and there was no red reflex.

This technique involved acute visualization of the intraocular structures never really seen before. No surgeon had ever really seen during surgery cortical material lying on top of a capsule or a tiny zonular dehiscence or a minute opening in the capsule, and yet this type of visualization was required if phaco was ever going to be successful.

The first microscopes I tried were tabletop dissecting microscopes, and they had inadequate side illumination. In examining other types of microscopes, I came upon an exciting discovery. Using an ENT microscope, the red reflex from the coaxial light gave me an incredible depth perception intraocularly. From then on, only ENT microscopes were used until Zeiss made one more suitable for ophthalmology.

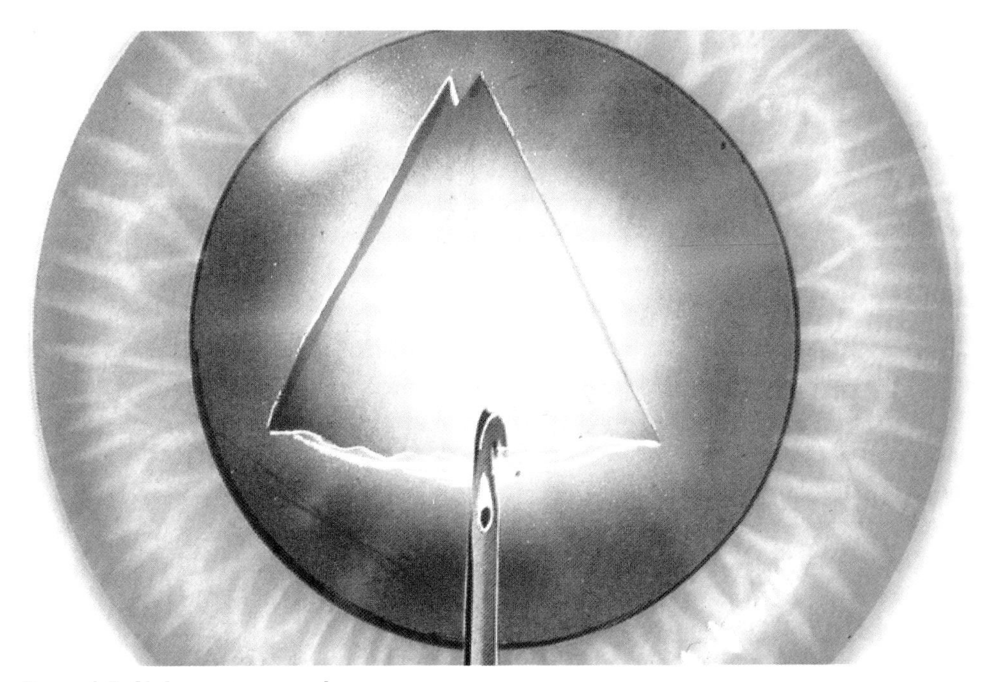

Figure 1-7. Christmas tree opening.

Protection of the Posterior Capsule

The posterior capsule is not a strong membrane. Techniques had to be developed that would protect it during the lens removal.

It became evident to me very early on that the big obstacle to phaco would be the rupture of the posterior capsule. The early phaco machines did not have the power or the suction that present models have, and the tip had to be pushed into a hard nucleus in order to emulsify it, like a dull knife must be pushed harder onto tissue than a sharp one. This pushing often broke the capsule. One must remember that there were no viscoelastics at this time. In order to make the procedure safer for me, and especially for others learning it, I devised a technique for prolapsing the entire nucleus into the anterior chamber, where it could be emulsified at some distance from the capsule. This method remained in vogue until the equipment was improved, at which time phaco in the posterior chamber (where phaco began) was reintroduced.

Protection of Iris and Cornea

A technique of surgery had to be developed that would allow the surgeon to safely emulsify the nucleus without damaging the endothelium or the iris.

In the early cases, the cornea collapsed many times against the vibrating needle, and the corneas had severe striate sometimes for up to 1 month. There was no method at this time of counting endothelial cells, but later studies showed up to 50% cell loss in these first cases. It is interesting to note that these corneas eventually cleared, giving the patients good vision.

Cortical Clean-Up

A technique would be needed to safely pull the cortex out of the fornices of the capsule, and then to aspirate it. In the early cases, the same phaco tip and sleeve were used to remove cortex, but it became obvious that this terminal opening endangered the capsule. I modified the tip, so that it had a closed terminal end, with the lumen on the side, so that it could be directed away from the capsule.

Instrument Problems

An instrument powerful enough to emulsify all types of cataracts without damaging adjacent structures would have to be developed.

The first phacoemulsifier used on animals and patients consisted of a table with various parts and devices connected to each other. One of the parts was a dental apparatus used to remove tartar from the teeth. This was modified so as to add suction and irrigation. The ultrasonic stroke was not only too small to act on hard cataracts, but it got dampened even further when a load (the cataract) was put on. I found that with piezo-electric crystals, rather than magnetostrictive stacks, a greater stroke could be achieved and dampening could be prevented. Today there is no cataract too hard to be emulsified.

Heat Build-Up

Ultrasonic frequencies build up sufficient heat to denature tissue. Cooling would have to be guaranteed.

After actually cooking and denaturing the protein of the lens in some animal eyes, it became clear to me that constant irrigation of the vibrating tip had to be assured. My original idea of having a water-tight, close-fitting incision was not going to work, since when the tip was occluded, the outflow through the tip was blocked, and since the incision was tight around the tip, no fluid could escape. It then became necessary to have the incision slightly larger than the tip so that fluid could always escape from the eye, and also to ensure that the amount of fluid flowing into the eye always exceeded the amount being aspirated. Once these concepts were put into effect, heat build-up ceased to be a problem.

Anterior Chamber Collapse

Considerable suction was necessary to hold lens material onto the vibrating tip. Once this material was aspirated, in a few milliseconds, there was enough suction build-up to collapse the chamber. The result of this collapse was to see the cornea touching the vibrating tip, with the endothelium being emulsified. A method had to be found to prevent this.

In order for the lens material (especially if it is hard nucleus) to remain fixed to the tip while that tip is vibrating, a fairly high level of vacuum must be achieved. If we started with a high level of vacuum, copious amounts of fluid would always be entering and leaving the eye. Also, if the capsule or iris were inadvertently engaged, these tissues would be more susceptible to damage than if the suction were lower. It became obvious that a peristaltic-type pump could apply minimum suction until such a time as the tip became occluded; at that time the suction would rise, holding the lens material onto the tip while it was being emulsified. The problem created with this system was that as soon as the lens material became suddenly aspirated, the high level of suction in the system would collapse the chamber. For the first 50 or so cases, I had no other solution to this problem other than that of trying to anticipate the collapse, and just before the morcel would be aspirated, I would take my foot off the foot pedal. This was very ineffective, and many times during the first cases, the cornea would collapse onto the vibrating tip. Although I am sure that the endothelium was damaged, to my good fortune, these eyes always cleared after a few days, permitting me to continue developing the instrument and technique.

After much searching, I finally found a fluid control system that monitored flow in arteries by creation of an electrical current from the ions as they rushed through the arteries. I adapted this system so that the fluid flow through the aspiration line was monitored. When it stopped (tip occlusion), a valve was put into the alert position. Within a few milliseconds after flow started up again (aspiration of the morcel), this valve would open to the atmosphere, killing the suction. This was a very satisfactory system, and was used for several generations of phacoemulsifiers. After having suffered through hundreds of actual collapses on my first cases, I still remember the joy of seeing the tiny "beat" of the cornea, instead of a collapse, once the system was working.

Handpiece Design

The early handpieces were extremely heavy and cumbersome. The original procedures took up to 4 hours, with over 1 hour of ultrasonic time. A special three-dimensional parallelogram had to be invented and constructed to hold the handpiece.

Ophthalmic surgeons are used to tiny instruments that fit into the fingers. The original phaco handpiece was about the size of a large flashlight, and weighed almost a pound. I was willing to use it while I was developing the techniques, but I knew no one else would be willing. While looking for ways to make the handpiece lighter and smaller, I developed the three-dimensional parallelogram to hold the handpiece, with all axes of rotation around the incision (Figure 1-8).

The original handpiece was magnetostrictive, and had a frequency of 25,000 cycles. By substituting piezo-electric crystals for the heavy magnetostrictive plates, the size and weight were greatly reduced, and the frequency was raised to 40,000 cycles. I now had a handpiece that others might be willing to try.

Handpiece Heat Build-Up

The original handpiece was magnetostrictive and had to be water cooled. This cooling water had to be isolated from the sterile end of the handpiece.

The original handpiece was water cooled. Non-sterile water flowed in, around, and out of the magnetostrictive plates. The first handpiece had a set of O-rings to isolate this non-sterile water from the sterile irrigation fluid, but in one instance the O-rings failed, causing an infection. The interim solution was to add a second set of O-rings, but finally, when the piezo-electric crystal replaced the magnetostrictive, air cooling was sufficient and no O-rings were needed.

Flaking of the Tips

The original tips were steel, and flaking was a problem, with the possibility of leaving iron shavings inside the eye.

Titanium is a completely inert metal and is silent in tissue. It also is less friable

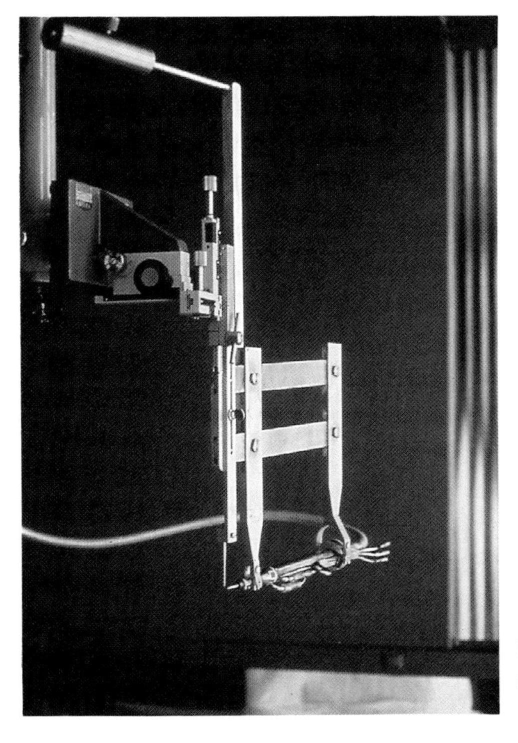

Figure 1-8. Three-dimensional parallelogram support for handpiece.

than steel, and therefore the steel tips were replaced with this metal, and in millions of cases now, there has not been any report of adverse effects from this material. It is extremely rare to see any particle in any operated eye.

Insulating the Vibrating Tip

The vibrating tip had to be insulated from the corneal scleral wound to prevent heating. Various materials were tried and the two best found were silicone and teflon. Since silicone was softer, it was the final choice.

Irrigating Solution

Since a fair amount of solution would be washing over the cornea during the procedure, it was important to find the best possible irrigating solution. Rather than embark on a scientific quest as to which solution would be the safest, I had observed in Barcelona that Joaquin Barraquer employed a solution, made in Spain, which closely approximated the fluid in the anterior chamber. I began importing and using this solution.

Political Problems

It is difficult enough for a serious scientist to introduce a dramatic change in a procedure that everyone thinks is already ideal. But when this new technique involves considerable training using an operating microscope when one has never used one before, when those who are unable to perform the new technique announce that you have to lose a "bucketful of eyes" before you are adept at it, and when that technique is developed by a saxophone player who is still appearing in Carnegie Hall and a comedian doing stand-up in the casinos of Atlantic City, it sounds like getting this procedure accepted would be a hopeless proposition.

At this point, I must say again, that if I had known in advance how many problems there were, I might never have started the project. The Chinese proverb is appropriate here: "The longest journey in the world begins with the first step."

Although the surgical and instrument problems outlined above were difficult to solve, they were a constant challenge and their solution brought a great deal of satisfaction. Not so for the political problems! When I first introduced phacoemulsification and aspiration, it was met with more than scientific reserve. It was met with scorn. How dare I, a young nobody, presume to change what the university professors were proclaiming the safest and most sophisticated surgical procedure ever devised (intracapsular surgery)? At meetings where I presented the concept, there was considerable derision, mockery, and hostility in the questions from the floor.

At the Manhattan Eye and Ear Hospital where I was assistant attending surgeon, the hospital voted to allow only one case per week, for every year an attending surgeon was on the staff. This vote cut down the number of cataract cases I could do. Since that edict affected only me, I was, after a great battle, able to get this ruling considered "restraint of trade," and the hospital had to withdraw that ruling. When I began doing phacoemulsification, the surgeon directors advised me that I would have to stop immediately if I had even one case of serious complications. When you put that sword of Damocles together with the problems outlined above with the technique and instrument, one can imagine the pressure involved in every procedure.

Once the technique had been taken up by several others in various parts of the country, each investigator was met with the same hostility that I had encountered. Once it began to be accepted by several dozen surgeons, the political forces against it had the operation declared "Experimental" by Medicare, meaning that there would be no reimbursement for the procedure. It took several months, and letters from a thousand patients from all over the country to get this ruling by the government reversed.

The American Academy of Ophthalmology then commissioned one of the most vociferous antagonists to the procedure to do an "unbiased" study comparing the results of phaco to intracapsular surgery. I was put on the panel, but was never allowed to see any of the results of this study until they were ready to be submitted. It came as no surprise to find that intracapsular surgery was found to be infinitely superior to phacoemulsification. Since the justification of this conclusion was rather suspect, I was able to engage the professor of statistics at Columbia Presbyterian University to examine the methods and conclusions drawn. His report was so scathing that the original report was discarded, and the final verdict submitted to the Academy was that phaco was at least as safe and effective as intracapsular surgery.

The increase in the percentage of cases done with phaco slowly increased over the years, until foldable lenses were introduced. At that time, phaco cases increased dramatically; today, phacoemulsification and aspiration are used to remove more than 85% of cataracts.

I am grateful to the early pioneers who stood with me, and grateful to all those who even today are improving this technique.

References

1. Kelman CD, Cooper IS. Cryosurgery of retinal detachment and other ocular conditions. *The Eye, Ear, Nose & Throat Monthly.* 1963;42:42-46.
2. Cryogenic surgery. *N Engl J Med.* 1963;268.
3. Kelman CD. Symposium: phacoemulsification. History of emulsification and aspiration of senile cataracts. *Transactions American Academy of Ophthalmology and Otolaryngology.* 1974;78:OP7-OP9.

Chapter 2

Alcon SERIES 20000 LEGACY Phacoemulsification System

I. Howard Fine, MD

Introduction

The SERIES 20000 LEGACY (Figure 2-1) is Alcon Surgical's sixth generation phacoemulsification system. It offers advanced design incorporating three dedicated microprocessors which control ultrasonics, fluidics, and the user interface, as well as a master computer that monitors and controls the overall system.

Ultrasonics

The ultrasonic driver is controlled by a dedicated microprocessor that allows for precise control of ultrasonic power at all power levels. The turbosonic handpiece itself uses a four-crystal transducer design whose benefits include:

- Stable power at any frequency or stroke.
- Stable power under varying load conditions.
- Multifrequency capabilities between 20 and 80 kHz.

Since the load, ie, the mass and density of nuclear material at the tip, is constantly changing, the system must be able to adapt to the changing conditions. If the system cannot, then the cutting efficiency will be compromised. Matching the driving frequency of the console with the operating frequency at the phacoemulsification handpiece is accomplished by a complex control system, "constant admittance tuning," which is new technology that enables LEGACY ultrasound handpieces to maintain optimal power regardless of cataract density. It allows the system to track ultrasonic frequency and power and provides real-time tuning at a sampling rate of 100 times per second.

The system provides an increased linear resolution of ultrasound power in a series of 1025 steps versus 265 steps in the previous Alcon system. This enhanced linearity, in 1% increments throughout the full range of ultrasound power, provides increased control over the full range of power including low-end power levels of phacoemulsification.

In addition to the new piezo-electric crystal configuration, there is a new computer-designed ultrasonic horn which provides increased cutting capability and efficiency as well as greater operative efficiency due to reduced heat output.

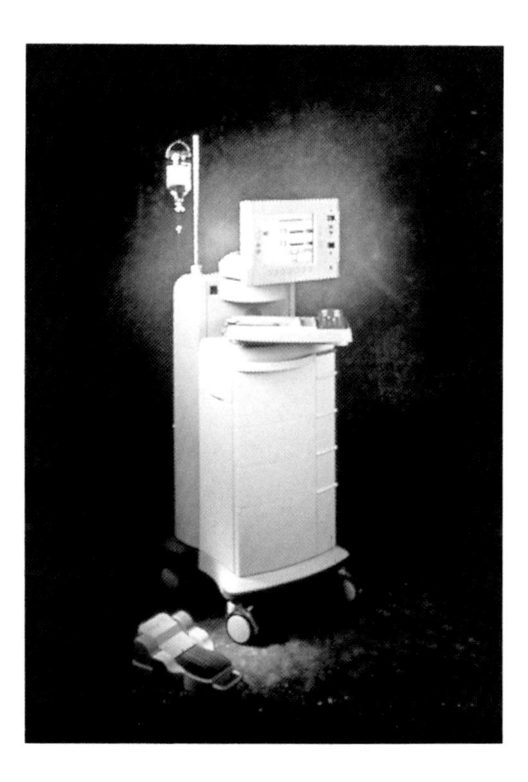

Figure 2-1. The Alcon SERIES 20000 LEGACY phacoemulsification unit.

The turbosonic tip is harmonically balanced to the ultrasonic handpiece. This enables optimization of the transmission of ultrasonic power to the turbosonic tip, producing more consistent and efficient cutting performance. In addition, the turbosonic tip allows for reduced acoustical positive pressure (Figure 2-2). Acoustical positive pressure is a forward wave of force that can repel nuclear material; the stronger the pressure wave the greater the vacuum necessary to overcome it. The turbosonic tip is aerodynamically designed to induce minimal resistance as it strokes through fluid. The effect of the design is the reduction of pressure waves, the enhancement of followability, reduced turbulence, and greater ability to achieve low and high vacuum techniques. The new hub design also eliminates the formation of bubbles.

The unique Kelman high-efficiency tip design, a new option, provides enhanced cutting and emulsification efficiency, enabling one to emulsify 4+ nuclei at lower power levels and, as such, facilitating phacoemulsification procedures which utilize sculpting or grooving for divide and conquer techniques. This system works because the unique configuration of the tip (Figure 2-3) provides a markedly enhanced cavitation phenomenon which allows for ablation of nuclear material in advance or in front of the tip without a need for contact of the nuclear material by

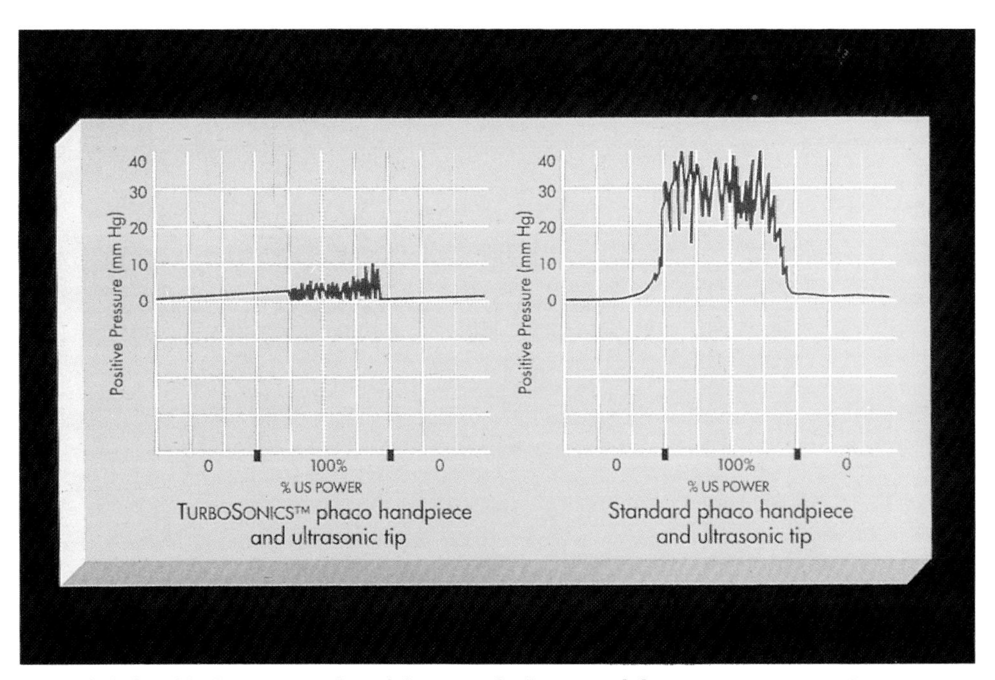

Figure 2-2. Graphical representation of the acoustical wave and the vacuum necessary to overcome it.

the tip itself. That is to say, in very hard nuclei one can actually create grooving and sculpting without any downward or forward force on the nucleus by the tip of the phacoemulsification handpiece. This is obviously an enormous advantage in cases of weakened zonules, zonular dialysis, pseudoexfoliation, post vitrectomy, and traumatic cataracts.

The tip and cap are covered by a more rigid sleeve to facilitate wound entry, to provide for improved thermoinsulation, and to resist inhibition of flow through the sleeve. The tapered hub also provides improved visibility (Figure 2-4).

Fluidic System

The fluidic system is controlled by a dedicated microprocessor that provides enhanced feedback and response. There is continuous monitoring of actual vacuum and precise control of fluid venting. This provides improved chamber maintenance and ensures rapid and controlled venting at all vacuum levels.

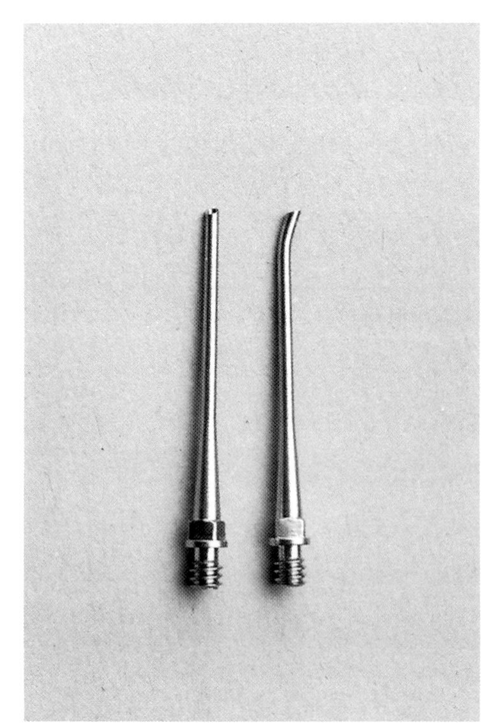

Figure 2-3. Comparison of the standard turbosonic tip to the left and the Kelman tip with a 30° bevel to the right.

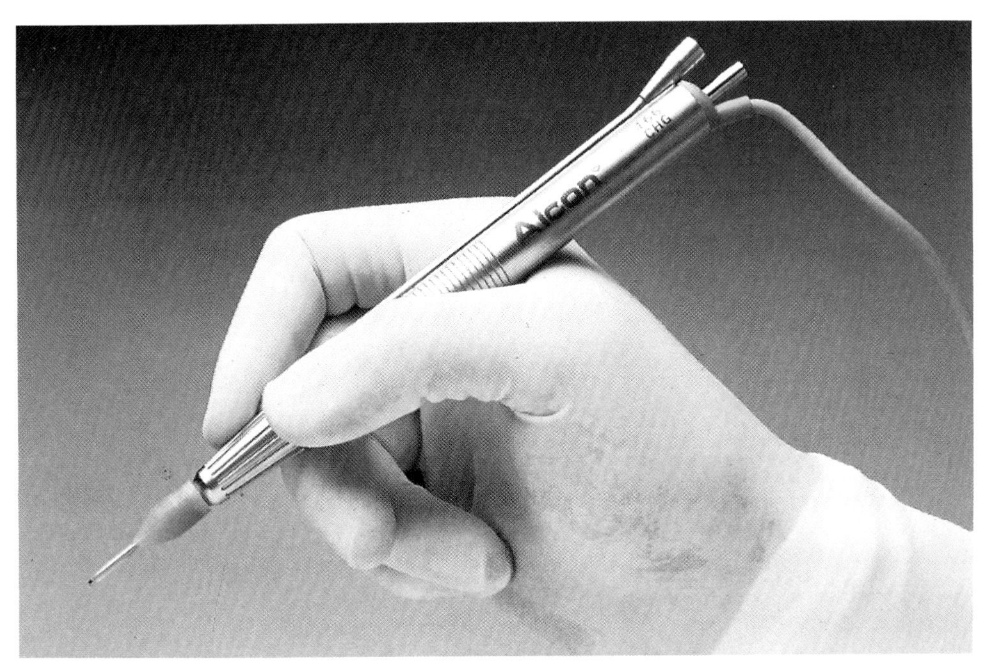

Figure 2-4. The assembled turbosonic handpiece with a Kelman tip.

In some systems, clearance of an occlusion at the phacoemulsification tip can result in a "surge" in which fluid from the higher pressure space, the anterior chamber, surges into the "negative" pressure space, the aspiration line connected to the phacoemulsification tip. If strong enough, the surge can cause posterior capsule vaulting and anterior chamber collapse.

Venting is the process whereby the negative pressure, or vacuum, is equalized to atmospheric pressure. In the SERIES 20000 LEGACY system a low compliance, liquid venting technique is used. Liquid venting utilizes irrigation fluid to neutralize the vacuum rather than air. Low compliance liquid venting is superior because fluid cannot be expanded or contracted, as air can, and thus fluid venting does not negatively affect fluidic performance. This system is also superior to reversing the pump, which can be associated with the introduction of air or contaminated fluid into the eye as well as the possibility of excessive pressure build-up. The digital control of the vacuum limit by the dedicated microprocessor provides precise control of the actual vacuum delivered to the eye and this enhances safety.

The new turbostaltic pumps are not as susceptible to compression related problems as are traditional peristaltic pumps because the turbostaltic pump (Figure 2-5) compresses the tubing around the pump head (Figure 2-6) rather than compressing

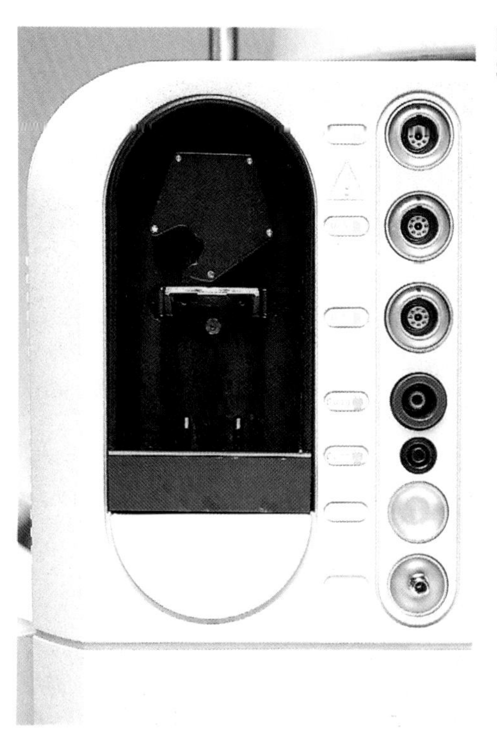

Figure 2-5. Five-roller floating head of the Alcon SERIES 20000 LEGACY pump.

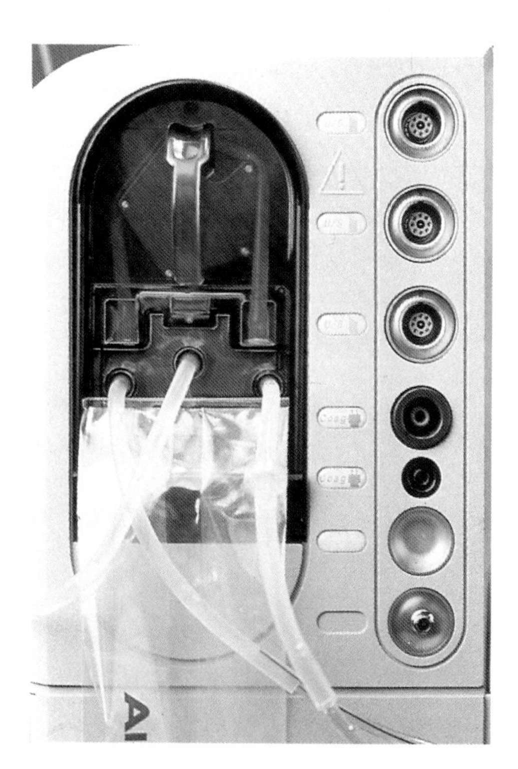

Figure 2-6. Cassette installed with the tubing drawn over the floating pump head, showing absence of compression from the outer side of the tubing.

it between two rigid surfaces. This reduces the pulsations to a nearly undetectable level and is a superior method for dampening pulsations compared to reducing the size of the tubing which restricts flow and requires higher vacuum to achieve equivalent flow rates. Small bore tubing introduces significant measuring error to the system and also reduces the possibility of low vacuum/low flow techniques. The advantages of the turbostaltic pump system are:

- The flow rate is determined by the speed at which the pump is turning.
- The vacuum will only build after occlusion has occurred.
- The rise time for vacuum is determined by flow rate.
- Vacuum will be reduced to pre-occlusion levels after the occlusion has broken.

Because of the non-compliant design very little potential energy is stored, vacuum levels can build regardless of flow rate, and rise time is predictable.

The turbostaltic system involves a microstepping pump motor, a five-roller pump head, a low compliance cassette, a floating cassette interface, and a dedicated microprocessor. Microstepping control of the pump motor allows the system to exercise very finite and accurate control of parameters such as vacuum rise time and aspiration flow rate. The five-roller pump head is geometrically balanced to provide optimal flow and minimal pulsations.

Design factors that were optimized to produce fluidic performance include the diameter of the pump head, number of rollers, distance between rollers, diameter of rollers, friction, tubing impression, and pinch force/duration. The cassette has been designed to be non-compliant by replacing much of the tubing with rigid molded fluidic channels which are integrated into the system (Figure 2-7). Rigidity of this design enhances fluidic responsiveness and the accuracy of control.

The floating cassette interface is achieved by having the tubing pulled around the pump head, floating freely rather than being compressed between rigid surfaces. The tubing can then absorb the pulsations generated by the peristaltic compression.

Compliance is the ability of an object to yield elastically when a force is applied. The more compliance that is designed into a fluidic system, the greater the impact on responsiveness and performance. Non-compliance is the ability of an object to maintain rigidity when a force is applied. The more non-compliant a fluidic system, the more responsive its performance will be. Non-compliant designs require more comprehensive control to compensate for the enhanced performance. Because air has elasticity and can be stretched or compressed, air venting systems introduce compliance into the aspiration line. Fluids, on the other hand, cannot be stretched or

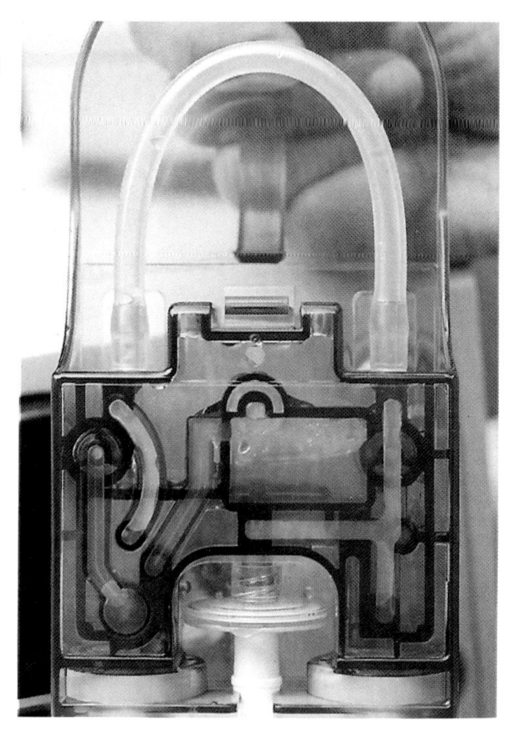

Figure 2-7. Pump cassette from the undersurface, showing molded plastic panels, eliminating tubing which thereby reduces compliance.

compressed and, as a result, fluid venting adds to the non-compliance of a system.

Microprocessor-controlled fluid venting achieves atmospheric pressure in the aspiration tubing at a rate calibrated to the levels of vacuum being built. Calibrated venting results in greater chamber stability, reduced chamber trampolining, elimination of water hammers, and reduced residual vacuum.

Flow rate has a very strong impact on fluidic performance and plays a significant role in determining rise time: the faster the pump speed, the faster the flow rate; the faster the flow rate, the shorter the rise time; the shorter the rise time, the better the followability. However, the shorter the rise time, the more susceptible the system is to surging and chamber instability if other fluidic variables and control systems cannot compensate as they do in this system.

Vacuum is also a variable in fluidic performance, but it plays a less important role. Any system can pull a vacuum if given sufficient time, more important is how fast the vacuum can be achieved and how the vacuum is controlled. If the vacuum is vented too rapidly and sharply, an overshoot condition occurs which causes the chamber to trampoline. Overshoot is a condition of alternating vacuum and pressure; if vacuum is vented incompletely then residual vacuum remains which can cause partial or complete chamber collapse. As in all peristaltic systems, the vacuum and flow rate can be set independent of each other.

The combination of new pump design with non-compliant cassette and microprocessor control has resulted in advanced fluidics with the advantages of both peristaltic and Venturi systems providing enhanced chamber stability and faster rise times.

User Interface

The system features a powerful central computer controlling three independent dedicated microprocessors. This provides the highest possible performance levels for control and monitoring the critical system functions of fluidics, ultrasound, and the control panel. The control panel with Ultratouch Screen Activation allows for easy and immediate access to all system functions. The front control panel rotates and tilts for maximum versatility and visibility with access for both the scrub nurse and the circulating nurse. The screen itself is a flat, 256-color, active-matrix, liquid crystal display which gives user-friendly icon graphical information, logically laid out for quick recognition with clarity and easy visibility (Figures 2-8 and 2-9).

The interactive interface provides a user-prompted, self-diagnostic, easy troubleshooting system with verification of data and a system of checks. The fully automated instrument set-up and breakdown includes a timing and tuning sequence with self-diagnostics. There is a purge of the system after each operation. There is a wireless, omni-directional remote control which allows access to all functions including bottle height, set-up and breakdown, memory access, mode change, and performance parameter adjustments. There is voice-confirmation technology which confirms changes of modes. This provides added levels of confidence and safety during surgery, reducing the possibility of user error and eliminating the need to check commands visually. There is extensive surgeon programmability, with a 96-memory option with 24 surgeon name custom programmability, instrument storage, and retrieval of custom programs. Each of 24 individual surgeons can have a four-memory option.

There is also a fully programmable multifunction linear control foot switch. Foot pedal modes include cautery, diathermy, reflux, and intraocular pressure control by adjustment of the IV pole height. Each of these functions can be brought into linear foot pedal control. The digital quadrature and coder technology utilized in the foot switch enhances control, comfort, and smoothness. This technology allows for cus-

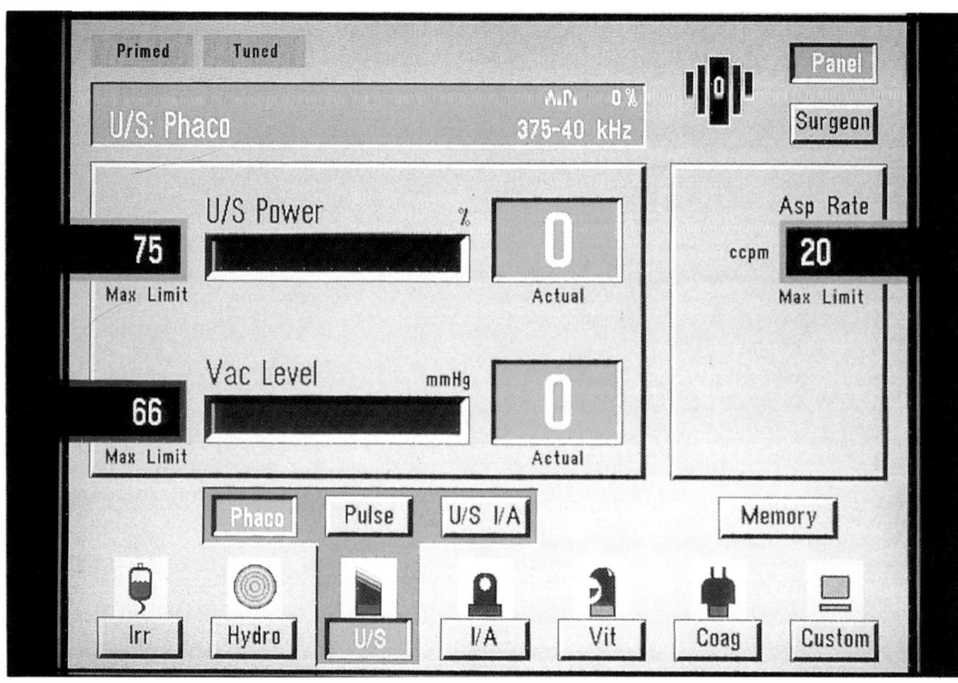

Figure 2-8. Example of one of the many possible user-friendly touch screens.

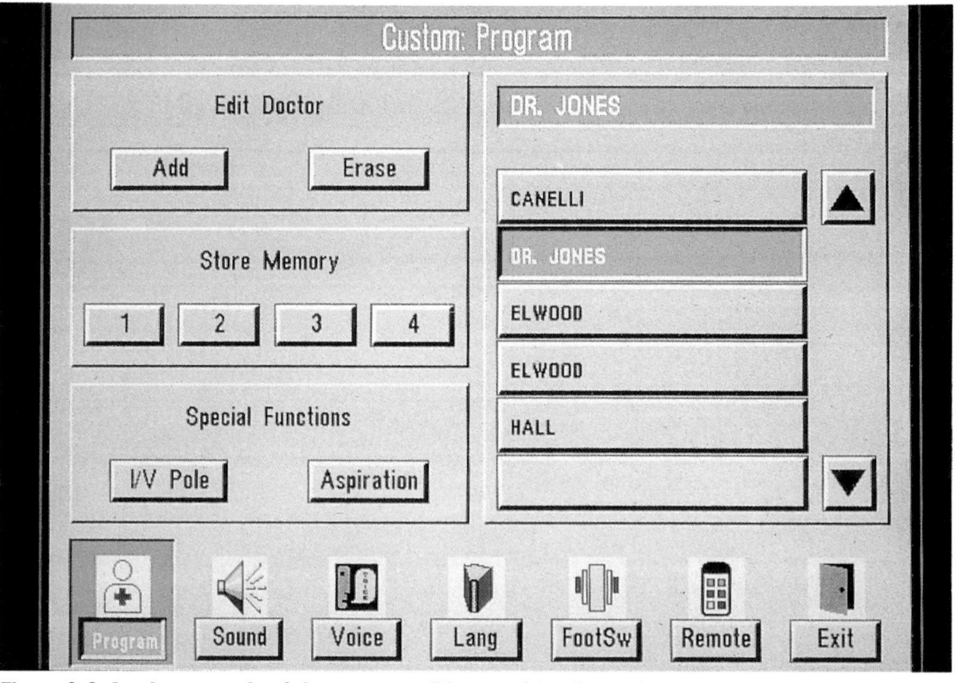

Figure 2-9. Another example of the many possible user-friendly touch screens.

tomized, detailed control of travel distance and tension for each foot position.

The Alcon SERIES 20000 LEGACY offers the phacoemulsification surgeon enhanced performance along with dramatic advantages in safety and control. This is achieved by microprocessor-controlled functions providing superior cutting efficiency, high performance fluidics with the advantages of **both** peristaltic and Venturi systems, and dramatically enhanced user-friendliness. Finally, the system has been designed to be easily and inexpensively upgraded with future developments.

The Surgical Procedure

The Alcon SERIES 20000 LEGACY provides cataract surgeons with a vast array of new options and capabilities which have allowed me to refine and enhance the various techniques I use during cataract surgery. With previous machines, it was difficult to alter parameters during surgery because the alteration process itself interrupted the procedure. However, the new programming capabilities provide a smooth transition from one set of parameters to another while retaining the enormous advantage of being able to set flow and vacuum independently.

Although I do chip and flip[1] for very soft nuclei and a variation of Paul Koch's stop and chop[2] for extremely hard nuclei, the procedure I use most frequently is crack and flip.[3] This procedure involves a 5-mm capsulorhexis, cortical cleaving hydrodissection,[4] hydrodelineation, and central grooving of the endonucleus into quadrants, without ever violating the epinuclear shell. This is followed by cracking, mobilizing the quadrants, trimming the epinucleus, and ultimately, flipping the epinucleus once its bulk has been reduced. Trimming and flipping the epinucleus is accompanied by mobilizing the cortex; in about 70% of cases, no cortex is left after removal of the epinucleus. In the other 30% of cases, I viscodissect the cortex into the capsular fornices and remove it along with residual viscoelastic after IOL implantation.

The programmability of the LEGACY allows customization of machine settings for each step of the procedure with modifications for different grades of nuclei. The foremost advantage of the LEGACY is the extremely efficient cutting capability at all power levels with lower turbulence and improved followability. This is the result of combining the redesigned handpiece, hub, and tip with the microprocessor-controlled, multifrequency, ultrasonic driver. With the Kelman tip one can groove extremely brunescent nuclei at low vacuum levels and a 16 mL/min flow rate without direct nuclear contact by the tip. As a result, there is no downward pressure on the nucleus and no forward movement—even without the second handpiece for countertraction. The expanded cavitation wave breaks the nucleus prior to contact by the phacoemulsification tip. This is particularly advantageous for cases characterized by weak zonules where there is increasing tendency throughout the procedure for retroplacement of the lens/iris diaphragm. Such cases can include patients with pseudoexfoliation, previous trauma, previous vitrectomy, and high myopia.

The advanced fluidics of this system are the result of a new pump design coupled with the non-compliant cassette and microprocessor control. These provide the advantages of both peristaltic and Venturi systems with enhanced chamber stability and faster rise times. Fluid venting is at the actual vacuum level within the anterior chamber, enhancing chamber stability. In many instances, this allows adequate chamber and posterior capsule stability for removing residual cortex with the phacoemulsification handpiece, without the threat of capsule rupture or vaulting.

The programmable features of the system allow the surgeon to have a different program for each grade of nucleus: soft, medium, and firm. Within each program there are four memory settings, one for each segment of the procedure: sculpting, quadrant removal, trimming of epinucleus, and flipping and removing the epinucleus. As can be seen in the machine settings parameter chart (Table 2-1), I do sculpting at zero to 6 mmHg vacuum with a flow of 16 cc/min. Quadrant (or chip) removal then takes place with a vacuum between 80 to 120 mmHg, depending on nuclear density. Trimming of epinucleus is done at 100 mmHg of vacuum. The vacuum is then reduced for flipping the epinucleus and removing the epinuclear shell. This allows new, reproducible levels of safety and control.

I use a new option, continuous irrigation regardless of foot position (see Table 2-1), as well as pulsed phacoemulsification, as soon as either grooving or sculpting has been completed. This means that as soon as there are mobile portions of nucleus in the eye, the balance of forces between the repulsive effect of the vibrating needle and the attractive effect of flow shifts in the direction of increased followability. Bottle height is set at 70 mmHg and the flow is maintained at 16 cc/min, which I find adequate for stable chamber depth and incision cooling.

This is an extremely user-friendly system. The multiple screens have easy-to-read icons and a continuous parameter display. The parameter readings on the screen change throughout the procedure and there is audio as well as visual confirmation of change in memory settings. As a result, the surgeon doesn't have to look at the screen or ask assistants to verify setting changes.

Use of the SERIES 20000 LEGACY has led to an evolution in my technique. I've switched to low-vacuum sculpting (between zero and 6 mmHg) and sweeping (HV

Gimbel, personal communication, March 1995) which allows me to rapidly develop a pattern of deep grooves in the endonucleus of extremely hard nuclei (Figure 2-10), or to make an initial groove and crack prior to using chopping techniques. Quadrant mobilization is characterized by a higher vacuum level with elevation of the apex of the quadrant and an ability to consume it with phacoemulsification-assisted aspiration while using the second handpiece to hold it within the epinuclear shell (Figure 2-11), maximally protecting the corneal endothelium. **Lower** phaco powers are used with **harder** nuclear fragments to keep the fragments/quadrants at the tip without chattering. Following quadrant removal, I trim the epinucleus. As the epinuclear rim is being trimmed, the precise settings (see Table 2-1) enable me to see cortex sweeping around the rim of the epinucleus and entering the phacoemulsification needle, without threatening the capsule and fornix or removing more of the epinucleus than desired. After three fourths of the epinuclear rim and roof have been removed, I switch to the flip memory at a lower vacuum. This allows controlled tumbling of the shell, removing it from its proximity to the capsule (Figures 2-12 and 2-13). Then,

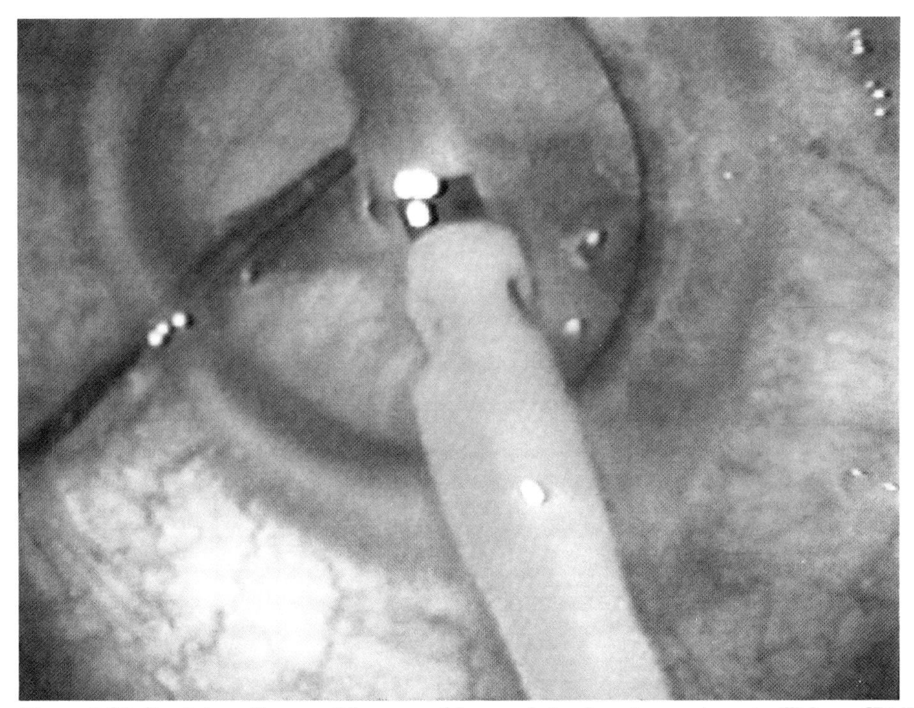

Figure 2-10. Cruciate pattern rapidly grooved in a rock-hard, mature cataract utilizing a 45° Kelman tip.

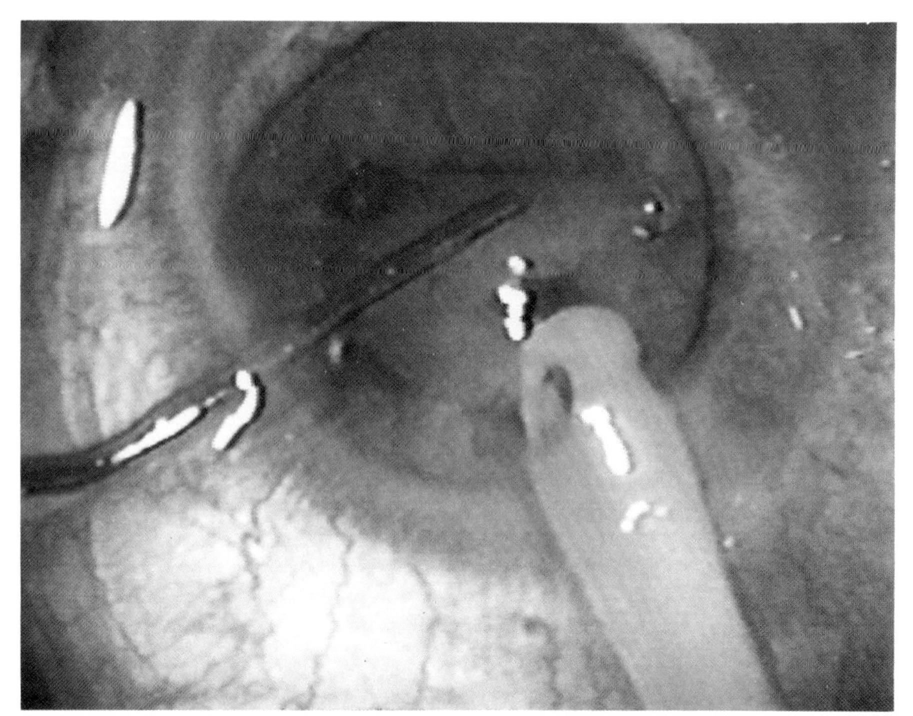

Figure 2-11. Removing the quadrant entirely within the epinuclear shell.

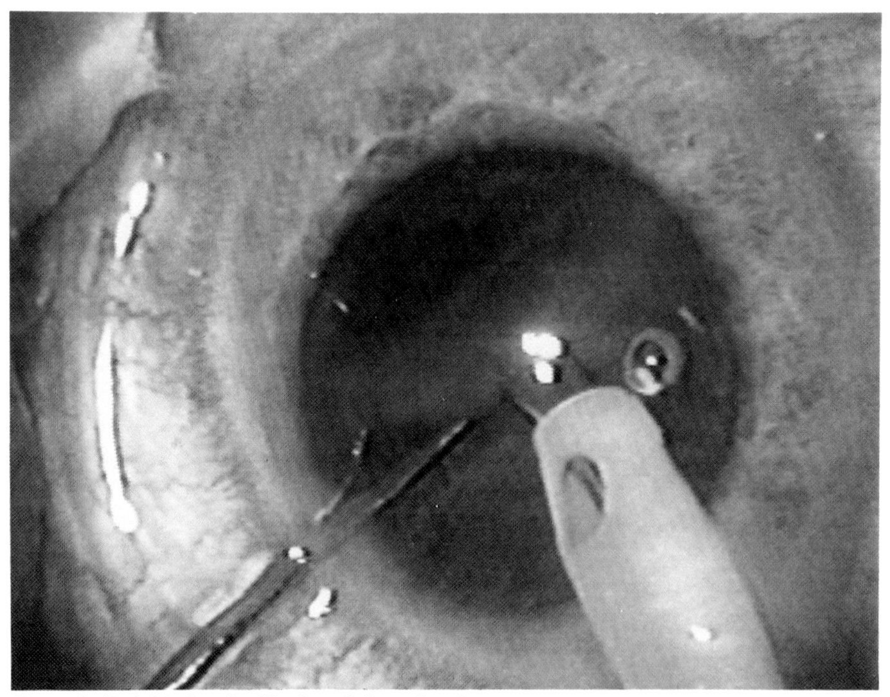

Figure 2-12. Initiating the flipping of the epinucleus.

with low powers of phacoemulsification or aspiration alone, I remove the epinucleus.

One of the most user-friendly features of the Alcon SERIES 20000 LEGACY is that there are three programs with up to six settings for each program. Surgical assistants can verify the grade of the nucleus prior to surgery and set the appropriate program before the surgeon enters the operating room. The surgeon may then simply call out the stage of the procedure, rather than a particular memory setting number. For example, he or she can simply say "Now grooving," rather than "Set at memory 1."

The procedure is divided into discreet, separate, highly reproducible steps, thereby increasing safety, control, and predictability. Altering the settings allows uniformity of technique on all grades of nuclear density. As the steps become more standardized and reproducible, there is increased efficiency in surgery, with reduced operating time and enhanced outcomes (Figure 2-14).

Foot position functions and Alcon LEGACY settings for vitrectomy procedures are shown in Tables 2-2 and 2-3.

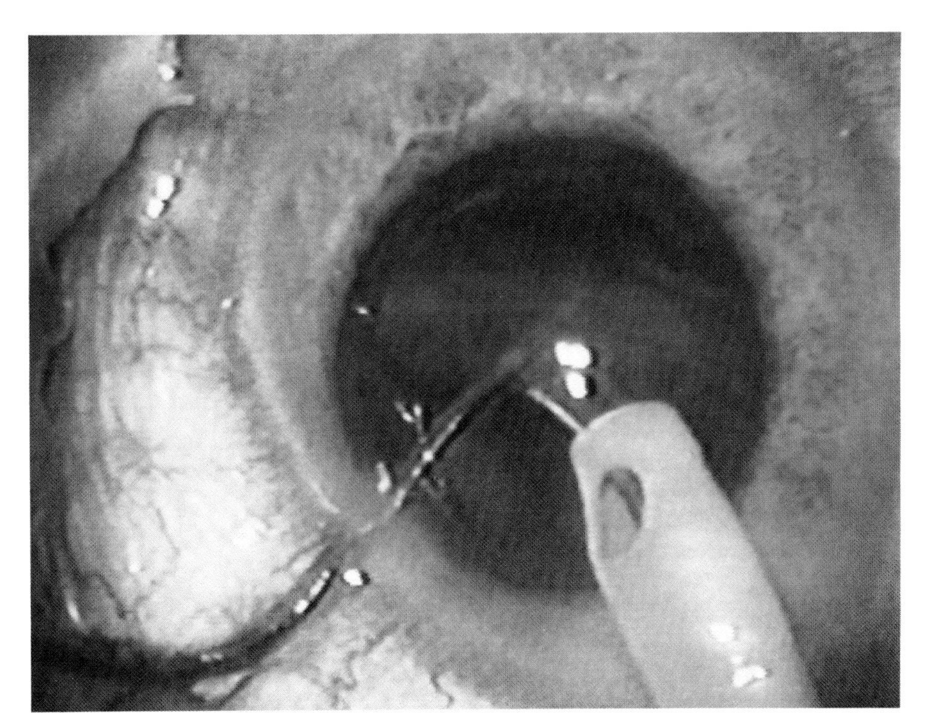

Figure 2-13. Near completion of the flipping of the epinucleus.

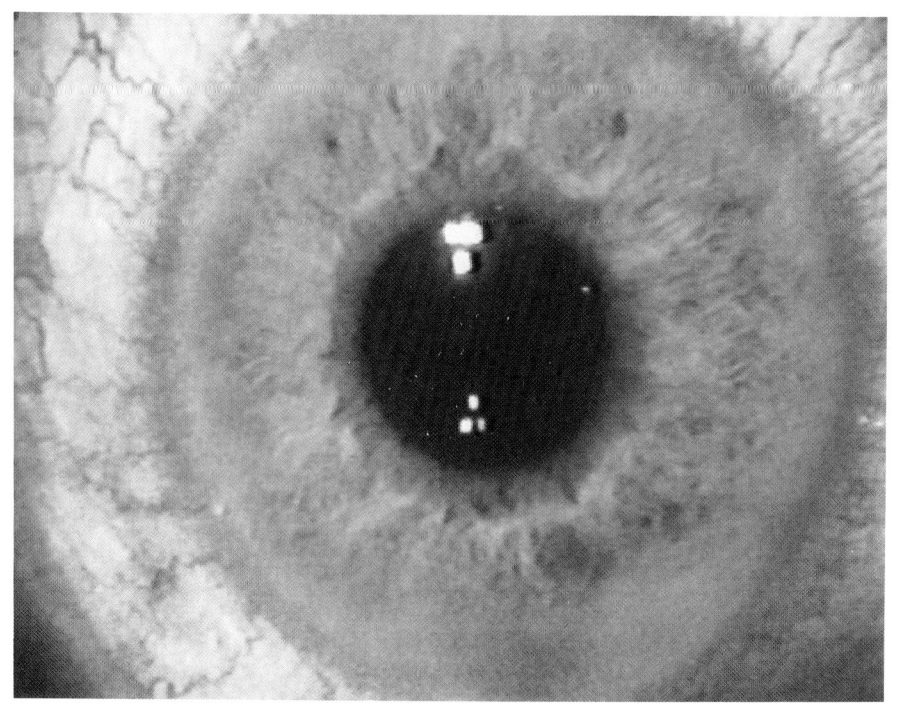

Figure 2-14. Immediate postoperative eye following phacoemulsification of a rock-hard, mature cataract with an IOL implanted.

Table 2-1. Fine Phacoemulsification Parameters with Kelman Tip

	Phaco Settings				I/A Control	
	Sculpt	Chip/Quad	Trim	Flip	Cortical Clean-Up	Viscoat Removal
	U/S Mem 1	Pulse Mem 1	Pulse Mem 2	Pulse Mem 3		
Power (Surg)	80	50-70	50-70	50-70	Surg Vac Control	
Asp/Flow Rate	12	16*	16*	16*	16*	30
Vacuum	0-6	80/100/120**	100	50	500	500
Mode	Cont	Pulse 8/sec	Pulse 8/sec	Pulse 8/sec	I/A Mode	I/A Mode

*Continuous irrigation.
**Nucleus 1-2+/3+/4+.
Bottle height=70cm.

Table 2-2. Foot Position Functions for Vitrectomy Modes

Foot Position	ATIOP	I/A Cutter
1	Irrigation	Irrigation
2	Cutter	Vacuum
3	Vacuum	Cutter

Table 2-3. Alcon LEGACY Vitrectomy Settings*

	Vitreous and Cortex Removal (no nuclear fragments)		Vitreous and Nuclear Fragment Removal	
Mode N1	Vit ATIOP	Vit I/A Cutter N4	I/A Cutter N4	Ranges
Vacuum	200-500	200-500	400-500	0-500
Asp/Flow Rate N2	30-60	30	30-60	0-60
Cut Rate	300	300	150-180	0-400
Port Size N3	0.5	0.5	0.9	0-0.9
BT HT	20-40	20-40	20-40	0-78

*Henry Mitchell, personal communication, June 1995.

N1=Irrigation tubing is attached to side-port cannula.

N2=Continuous flow irrigation can also be selected.

N3=The port size can be adjusted by holding the back of the ATIOP handpiece and turning the gray wheel left or right. Do not hold the handpiece by the irrigation sleeve—it will turn freely around the cutter blade shaft. The best procedure for adjustment is done under the scope. Do not activate the cutter out of fluid. This will dull the blade! Adjust the port size smaller for cortex removal and increase vacuum to 300 to 400 mmHg. Adjust the port size larger for nucleus removal and increase vacuum to 400+ mmHg. Also adjust cut rate to 150 to 180 cuts per minute.

N4=Settings must be programmed into memory.

References

1. Fine IH. The chip and flip phacoemulsification technique. *J Cataract Refract Surg.* 1991;17:366-371.
2. Koch PS, Katzen LE. Stop and chop phacoemulsification. *J Cataract Refract Surg.* 1994;20:566-570.
3. Fine IH, Maloney WF, Dillman DM. Crack and flip phacoemulsification technique. *J Cataract Refract Surg.* 1993;19:797-802.
4. Fine IH. Cortical cleaving hydrodissection. *J Cataract Refract Surg.* 1992;18:508-512.

Chapter 3

Phacoemulsification with the Allergan Medical Optics Prestige Phacoemulsification Unit

Roger F. Steinert, MD

The Allergan Medical Optics Prestige Phacoemulsification Unit evolved from the desire to optimize the matching of a surgeon's operative goals with the mechanical performance of the phacoemulsification unit. Phacoemulsification cataract surgery presents a wide range of conditions; safety and efficacy of the procedure can be achieved only with a flexible and responsive device that works harmoniously with the surgical style of the physician.

In this chapter, we will review the essential surgical goals of phacoemulsification cataract surgery, the design goals of the AMO Prestige Unit, the distinction between "powerful phacoemulsification" versus "phacoemulsification power," the features and benefits of the AMO Prestige Unit, and my personal experience with the Prestige device.

Surgical Goals

Small-incision cataract surgery requires **disassembly** of the nucleus. Disassembly of the nucleus requires the input of **energy**.

In small-incision cataract surgery today, potential sources of energy are ultrasound, a second instrument, vacuum, and irrigation. Future cataract surgery may add energy input with laser light. These sources of energy are listed in Table 3-1.

Ultrasound energy radiates from the source, with the potential for collateral tissue damage. Uncontrolled irrigation causes turbulence, and particles within the fluid may damage vulnerable cells, particularly the endothelium, as well as potentially lacerate the fragile posterior capsule. In contrast, the second instrument and vacuum are **locally contained** energies. Properly employed, these energy sources are inherently safer. Bimanual phacoemulsification began with the simple goal of facilitating favorable presentation of the nucleus to the phacoemulsification tip through the tilt maneuvers pioneered by Richard Kratz. Surgeons then realized that the second instrument could actively participate in the disassembly of the nucleus, in the nuclear fracturing techniques taught by Howard Gimbel and John Shepherd.

Until new technology that now permits the utilization of high levels of vacuum, however, surgeons have not had access to this second source of energy. High vacuum improves ultrasonic coupling by holding the nucleus tightly to the phacoemulsification tip. This tight coupling enhances the efficiency of the ultrasonic destruction of the hard nucleus. Moreover, the vacuum itself can fragment the nucleus, as a rigid nuclear chip is pulled into apposition against the phacoemulsification tip, fracturing the nucleus into smaller particles. Finally, high vacuum is capable of aspirating larger chips, reducing the need to use more ultrasonic energy to create nuclear "dust" or emulsate. Table 3-2 summarizes these three contributions of high vacuum. Through each of these three mechanisms, total ultrasonic energy requirements are reduced. The nuclear disassembly procedure becomes one of "phacoaspiration" more than "phacoemulsification."

Moderate flow rates are an important adjunct to high vacuum. It is the flow of BSS that brings nuclear fragments to the ultrasonic tip. The irrigant flow is an important element in cooling the phacoemulsification tip. Finally, flow is needed to clear nuclear chips from the aspiration line.

Design Goals of the AMO Prestige Unit

The AMO Prestige Phacoemulsification Unit, shown in Figures 3-1A through 3-1D, was designed in consultation with leading cataract surgeons as an innovative

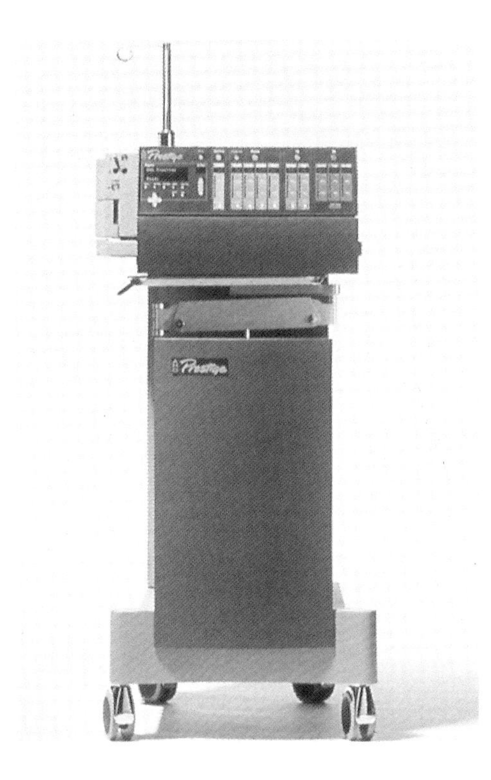

Figure 3-1A. The AMO Prestige Unit with independent stand and integrated motorized pole for BSS infusion.

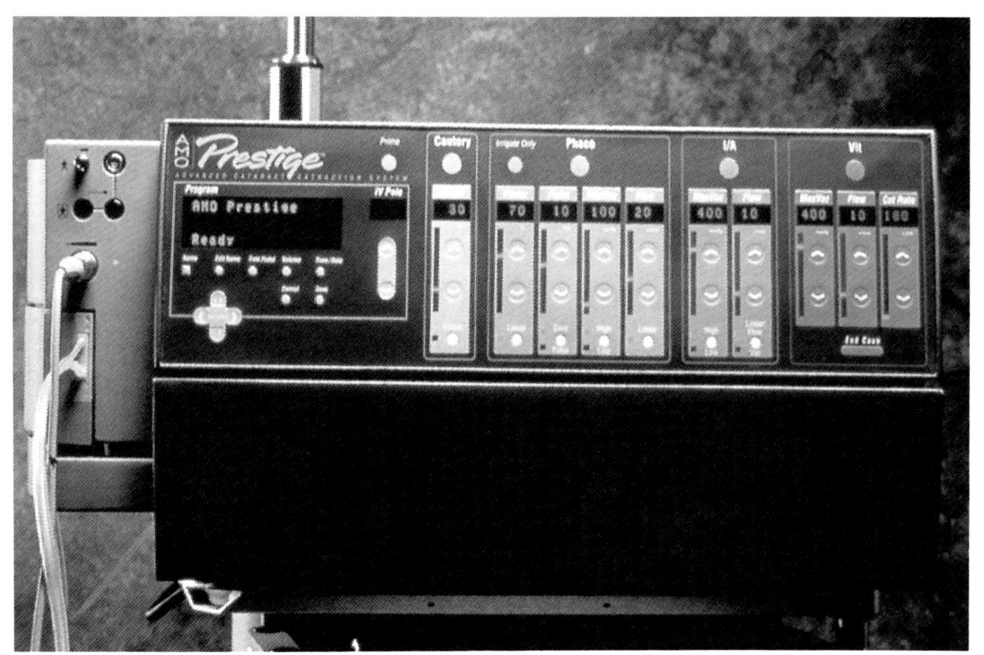

Figure 3-1B. The control panel is intuitive, user-friendly, and provides precise control over all aspects of phacoemulsification.

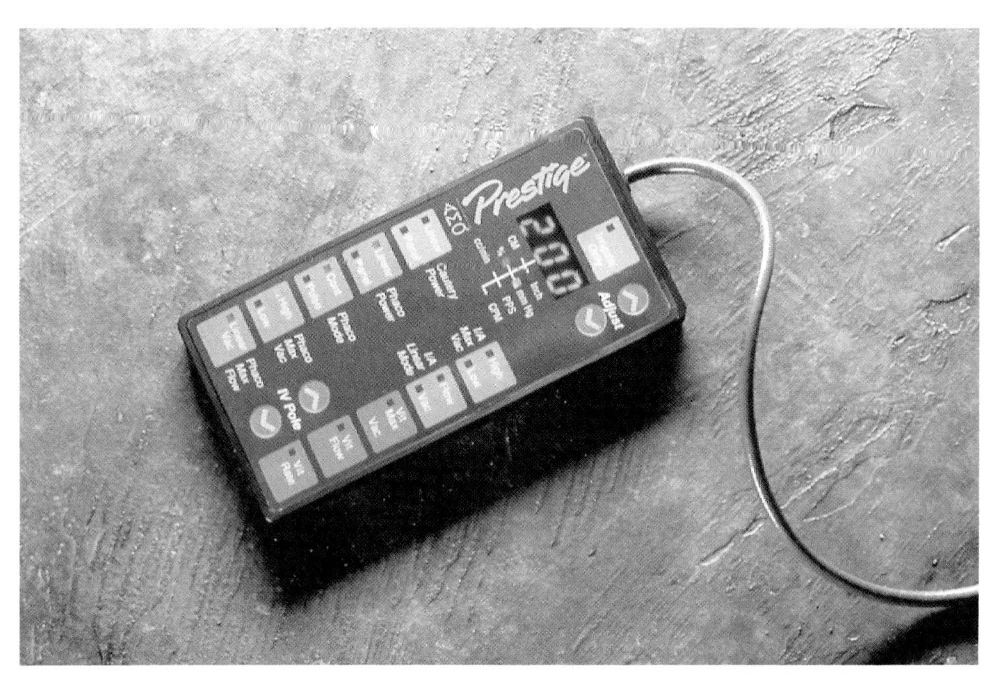

Figure 3-1C. The remote control allows separate input of all important variables from the sterile instrument tray.

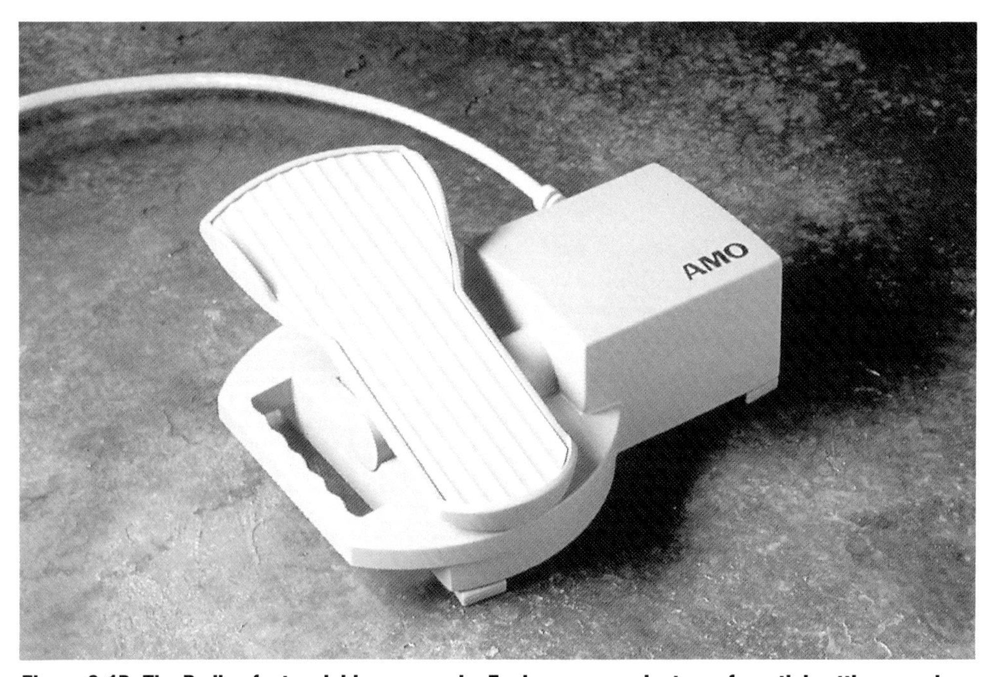

Figure 3-1D. The Radian foot pedal is ergonomic. Each surgeon selects preferential settings, such as the range of travel for each function.

device that would meet the three principal needs unmet by existing phacoemulsification technology.

The first requirement was reduction of ultrasonic energy required to complete the procedure, utilizing flow and vacuum as key components in the removal of the cataract.

Second, surgeons desired a flexible device, providing the rapid response traditionally associated with Venturi systems while maintaining the safety and flexibility of peristaltic systems, with the ability to independently set aspiration and vacuum levels.

The third goal was a user-friendly device that is intuitive, allowing each user to easily set up and subsequently customize the parameters of the machine to maximize an individual surgeon's preferences. The unit must be able to accommodate changing levels of surgical skill, variable intraocular conditions, and different types of cataract. Table 3-3 summarizes these design goals.

The design goals of the AMO Prestige Unit were therefore to provide surgeons with an innovative device that would meet the needs of surgeons to perform a wide range of current and future phacoemulsification surgical techniques, simultaneously delivering a safe and stable intraocular environment under a variety of conditions.

"Powerful Phaco" Versus "Phaco Power"

With the growth in popularity of phacoemulsification over the past two decades, the emphasis for surgeons has been on learning to use ultrasound energy to destroy the nucleus in a controlled manner. Fluidics have either been completely ignored or, at best, an afterthought. Surgeons now increasingly appreciate that fluidics of a phacoemulsification system are a critical environmental element that must be optimized in order to improve both the versatility and safety of the procedure. The surgeon desires **powerful phacoemulsification**; fluidic safety and control offer powerful phacoemulsification without resorting to deleterious levels of raw **phaco power**. To draw an analogy to the automotive world, this is the difference between driving a highly but proportionately powered sports car with an equally fine-tuned chassis down a winding road, compared to negotiating the same course in a sedan with a sloppy suspension but a "souped up" engine.

Table 3-4 reviews the advantages and disadvantages of using high levels of phacoemulsification energy for cataract extraction, while Table 3-5 lists the benefits and drawbacks of low energy phacoemulsification surgery.

Surgeons need to minimize the use of raw phacoemulsification power, yet still benefit from a "powerful phacoemulsification system." Table 3-6 describes the behaviors of such a truly powerful system.

The design challenge is to conceive and produce the components that allow a powerful yet safe system. To attract the nucleus and achieve good "followability," one needs a moderately high level of inflow and outflow under conditions where there is no occlusion. To hold the nucleus, however, one needs high vacuum when occlusion of the tip occurs. Smooth emulsification of the nucleus requires a sophisticated microprocessor-controlled phacoemulsification handpiece with high frequency oscillation and high tip acceleration, yet exquisite surgeon control. Stability of the anterior chamber requires controlling fluidics under all conditions of cataract surgery, and most importantly, defeating the dreaded "post-occlusion surge" phenomenon.

Post-occlusion surge occurs due to the build-up of potential energy when the phacoemulsification tip is occluded and vacuum builds within the aspiration line. As illustrated in Figure 3-2, vacuum within the flexible aspiration tubing causes an invisible yet significant compression of the tubing by the negative internal pressure compared to outside atmospheric pressure. Moreover, any gas bubbles in the aspiration line expand under vacuum conditions, just like an elongated spring. At the moment when the occlusion of the phacoemulsification tip clears, the vacuum in the aspiration line drops to zero. The tubing immediately expands to its original diameter, increasing the internal volume of the aspiration line. Expanded gases contract, just as a stretched spring pulls back. This also expands the effective internal volume of the aspiration line. These two forces cause the internal volume of the aspiration line to increase, and this volume must be met by fluid drawn from the anterior chamber. If this volume cannot be met by the volume of infusion fluid in excess of wound leakage, then the posterior capsule comes forward and the corneal dome collapses as anterior chamber volume is diminished (Figures 3-3A through 3-3G).

Surgeons have traditionally dealt with post-occlusion surge in several ways. The maximum vacuum employed is reduced to "safer levels," sacrificing the advantage of high vacuum at other times in the procedure. Similarly, aspiration rate is also decreased, at the sacrifice of followability. Infusion is improved by raising the bottle and tightening wounds. Finally, the surgeon learns to anticipate post-occlusion surge by lifting the foot off the pedal when a fragment begins to be aspirated into the phacoemulsification tip. If the surgeon is a little too eager, however, the procedure is interrupted and the fragment remains at the phacoemulsification tip. If the surgeon is a little too slow, then the post-occlusion surge hits with a vengeance, and

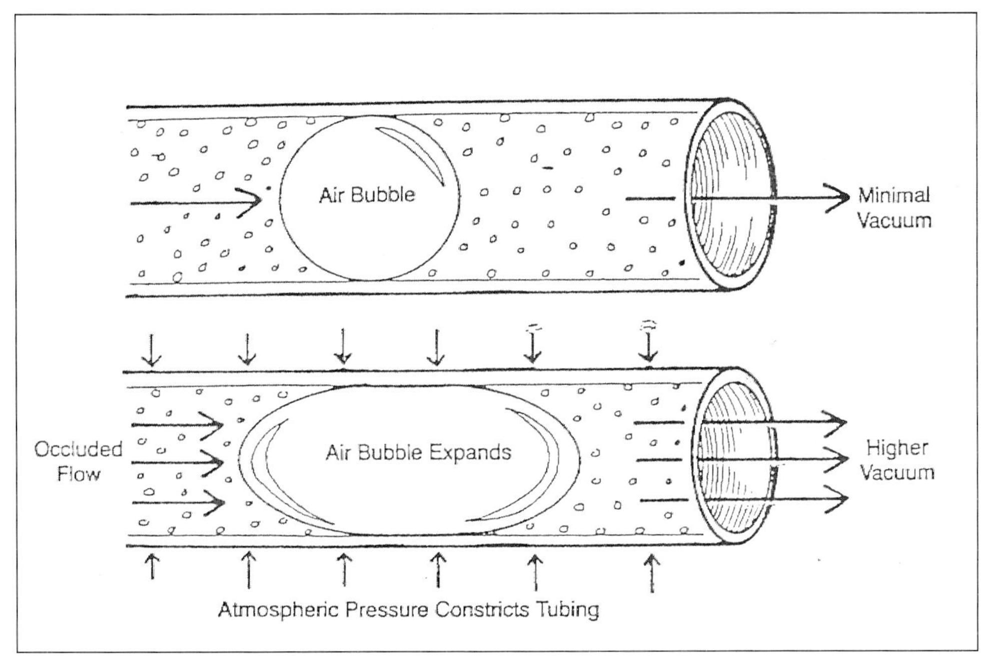

Figure 3-2. The effects of occlusion. When the aspiration line is occluded, generating higher vacuum levels, the pressure inside the tubing becomes lower than atmospheric pressure. The atmospheric pressure therefore constricts the tubing, and any internal air bubbles expand. This phenomenon stores potential energy within the system. When the occlusion is released, the reexpansion of the tubing to its normal diameter releases the potential energy, causing a momentary acceleration in the aspiration rate, clinically known as "surge." Reproduced with permission from Steinert RF. *Cataract Surgery.* Philadelphia, Pa: WB Saunders; 1995.

the posterior capsule may be aspirated into the phacoemulsification tip or the corneal endothelium damaged. Post-occlusion surge occurs whether the pump is peristaltic, Venturi, or diaphragmatic.

Figures 3-3A through 3-3F illustrate the flow and vacuum elements of normal phaco fluidics and post-occlusion surge.

Features and Benefits of the AMO Prestige Unit

The AMO Prestige features three characteristics:

- Advanced computer technology
- High-performance fluidics (ASET—Applied Stable Eye Technology)
- Other programmable features

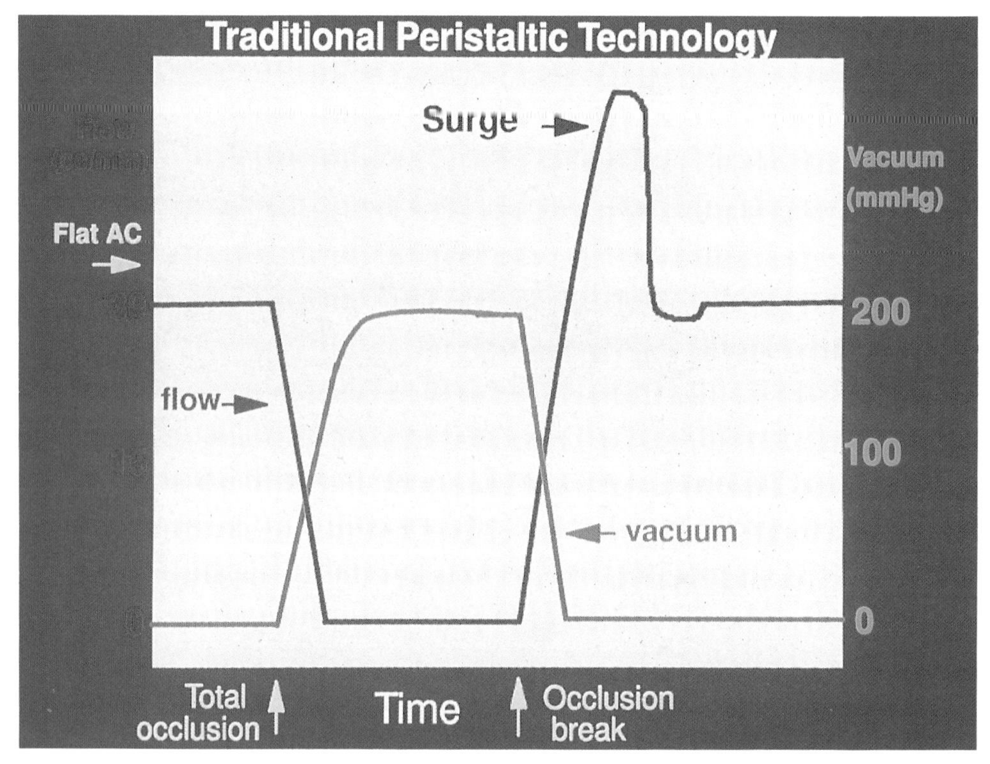

Figure 3-3A. The dynamics of vacuum and flow are graphed, with particular emphasis on the phenomenon of surge. The values shown are illustrative and not necessarily those of any particular commercial system or surgical technique. In traditional peristaltic technology, flow ideally can be set at a relatively high rate just below that which would flatten the anterior chamber. In a nonoccluded system, the flow is high, and the vacuum level at the phacoemulsification tip is nearly zero. When the tip is occluded, the aspiration rate rapidly falls to zero. The vacuum level rises correspondingly. The more rapid the flow rate, the more quickly the vacuum level rises. The vacuum level continues to build up to the preset limit, after which fluid is bled into the aspiration line, limiting the maximum vacuum. When occlusion is relieved, the vacuum then rapidly falls back to a near-zero level at the tip. The stored potential energy in the aspiration line causes a momentary "surge" in the fluid flow before the flow stabilizes at the original level. If the potential energy causes a surge of fluid flow greater than the combined rate of irrigation fluid inflow and wound leak, flattening of the anterior chamber results.

The combination of these features in one system allows the surgeon to safely experience benefits of both Venturi and peristaltic systems, and therefore revolutionize the technique of phacoemulsification surgery.

The microprocessor is the brain of this highly sophisticated system, driving the fluidics and other characteristics. The fluidics are controlled in the following way:

- The microprocessor monitors fluid pressure changes. It senses the formation or clearance of occlusions at the tip as well as any vacuum changes.

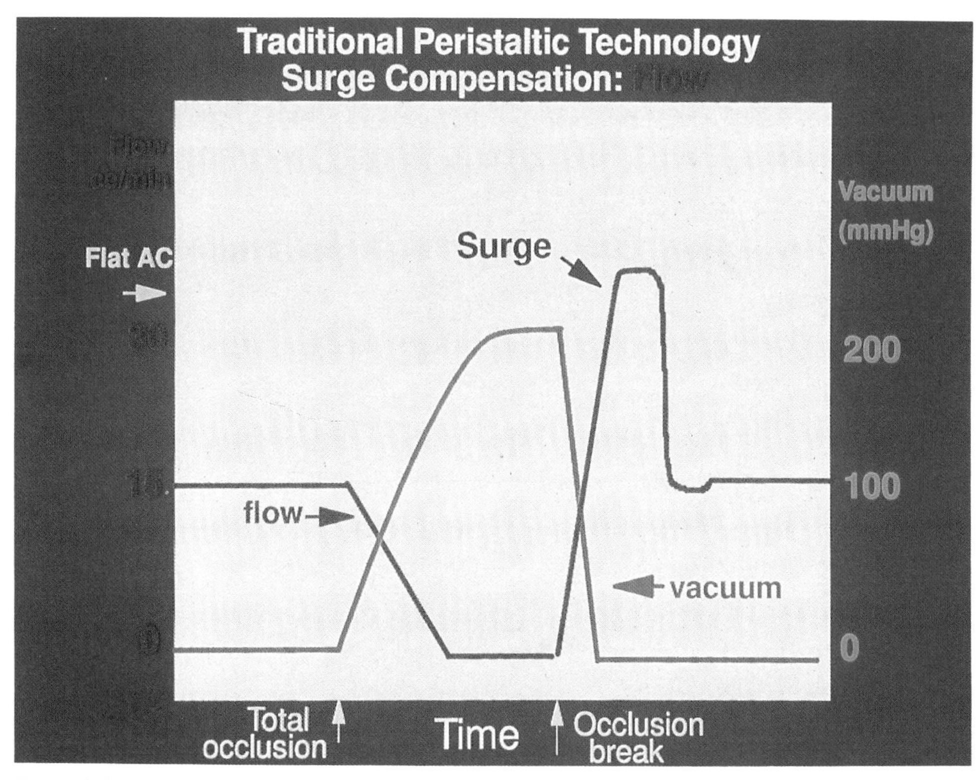

Figure 3-3B. One mechanism for compensating for surge is to reduce flow. When flow, or aspiration rate, is reduced, two effects are seen. First, after occlusion is obtained, the rate at which the vacuum rises is slower. Ultimately, however, the vacuum still builds to the preset level. Second, after occlusion break, the height of the fluid surge is the same as in Figure 3-3A. However, the surge is relative to the baseline level of nonoccluded flow. Because the flow has been reduced, the peak surge level may be at or below the level of a momentary flattening of the anterior chamber.

- As vacuum builds, the computer then modulates the pump speed to minimize pressure swings and post-occlusion vacuum surges which may cause AC dimpling and capsule motion.

This ultimately results in stability throughout the procedure, even at high vacuum levels.

The block diagram in Figure 3-4 shows the design concept and information flow with the various components of the AMO Prestige. This diagram illustrates how the microprocessor:

- Interacts with the mechanical aspects of the pump.
- Interacts with the surgeon's particular programmable settings and the system software to bring about the desired surgical result.
- Documents the surgical parameters and the machine performance through the printer.

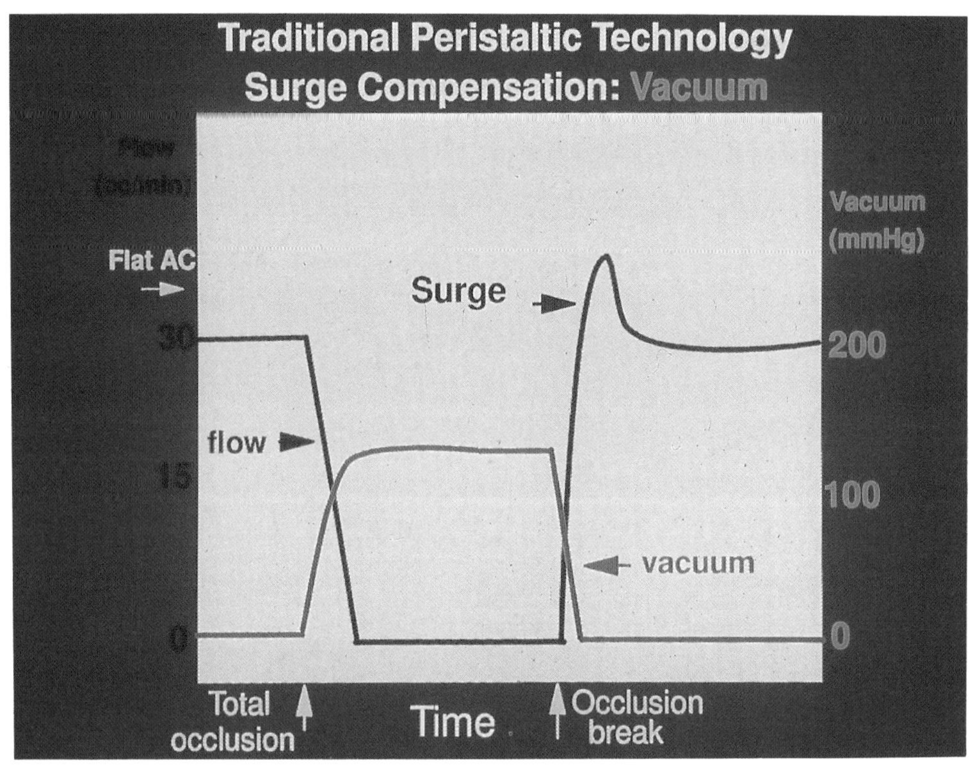

Figure 3-3C. An alternative compensation for surge is to reduce the vacuum level. Because the flow rate is unchanged, the speed at which the maximum vacuum is achieved is unchanged compared with the build-up of vacuum seen in Figure 3-3A. After the occlusion is relieved, the amount of surge is reduced because the stored potential energy is reduced because of the lower vacuum level. With high flow rate, however, even this reduced amount of surge may exceed the level at which flattening of the anterior chamber is seen.

It is the computer that:

- Finely tunes the handpiece and adjusts the frequency during the procedure.
- Stores machine settings, conditions used during the procedure, and a diagnostic history of the machine.
- Also handles multiple tasks such as priming the phaco handpiece while allowing the surgeon to use cautery.

The unique fluidic technology, which Allergan calls ASET for Applied Stable Eye Technology, describes how the software and hardware work together to provide stable, safe intraocular pressure even at high vacuum levels. The fluidics are microprocessor controlled. A model of the anterior chamber is established in the cartridge. The pump continuously adjusts its speed based upon feedback from the microprocessor, which reads the pressure in the anterior chamber model and senses the approximate pressure in the eye. Finally, the diameter of the aspiration and irriga-

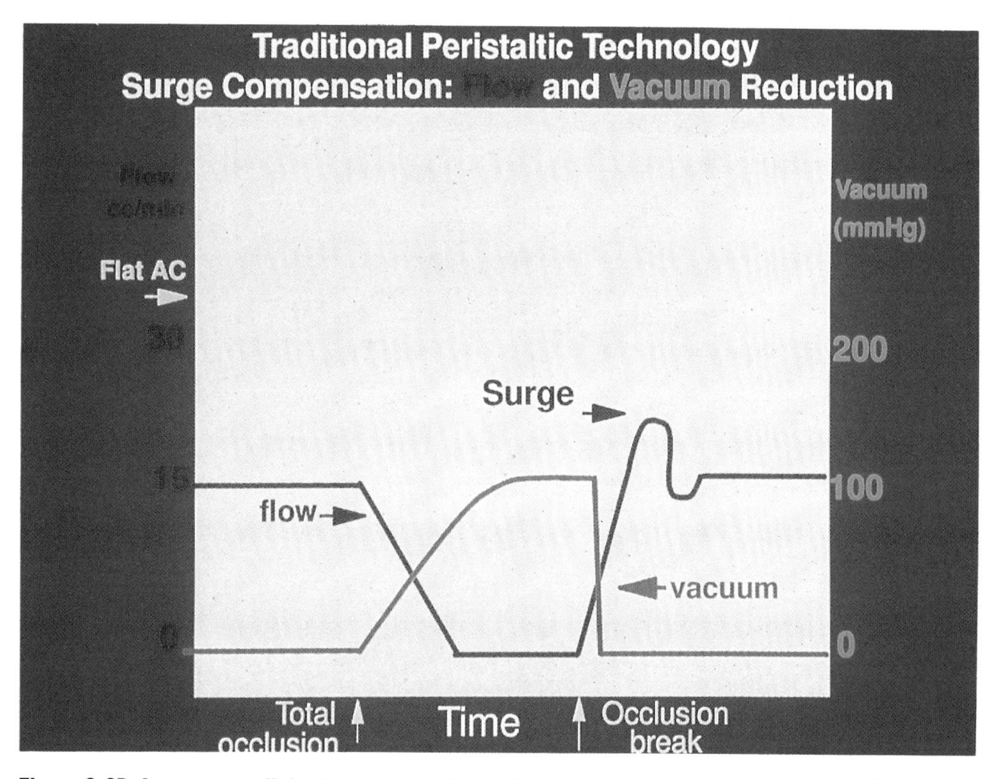

Figure 3-3D. In common clinical practice, both the flow and the vacuum levels are reduced below the theoretical maximum to guard against surge. As illustrated, the reduction in flow rate and maximum vacuum level reduce the peak surge below the level at which the anterior chamber flattens. Through these compromises, safe phacoemulsification can be clinically performed, but with marked compromise of the potential fluidic performance.

tion tubing has been optimized to provide a balanced inflow to outflow ratio.

Figure 3-3G demonstrates the elimination of post-occlusion surgery with ASET.

Other features were incorporated to enhance the versatility of the machine. The system's memory card, which contains the system hardware that governs the operation of important machine functions, is interchangeable and upgradable. This provides an efficient means of changing or adding machine features and enhancing/fine-tuning machine performance without the need to purchase a new machine or expensive hardware changes.

The Radian foot pedal can be customized by each surgeon for particular preferences (reflux switches, degrees of travel for each position, two- or three-step vitrectomy). The additional position in the three-step vitrectomy is an I/A mode only. The objective of adding this was to enable the surgeon to use the vitrectomy cutter as a substitute I/A handpiece in order to perform cortical clean-up in the presence of vitreous.

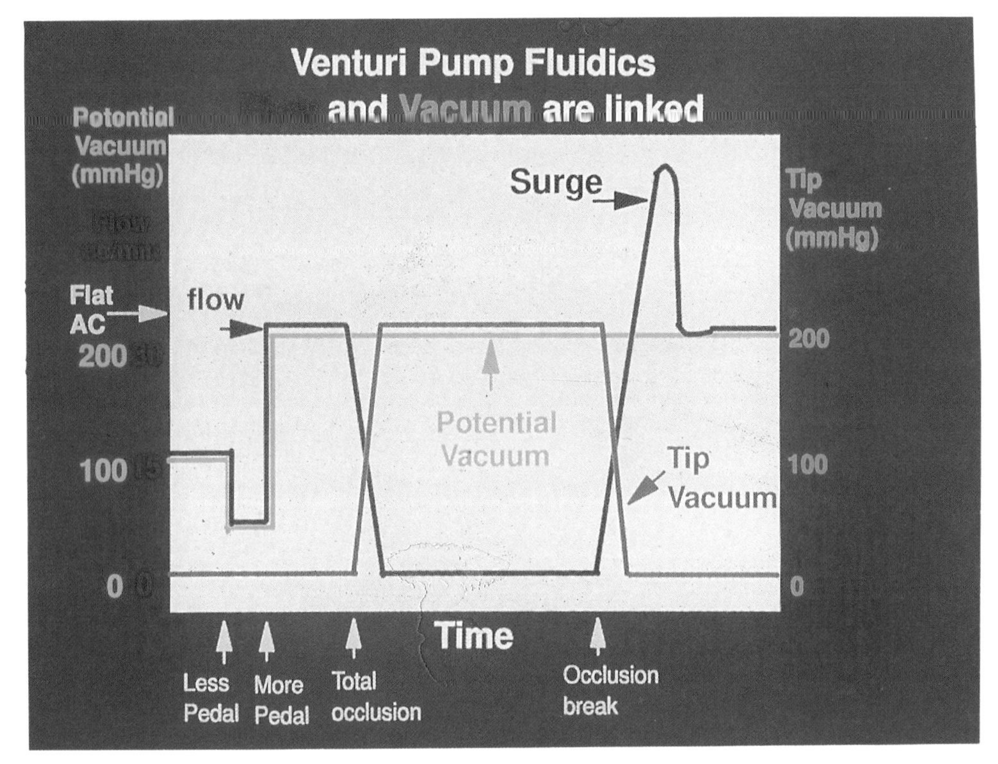

Figure 3-3E. In a Venturi or diaphragm pump, flow and vacuum are intrinsically linked. The potential vacuum within the system caused by the Venturi and diaphragm pump is the principal determinant of the flow level. As illustrated in the left side of this figure, one attribute of the traditional Venturi system is the rapid response time of the flow rate achieved by varying the potential vacuum within the system. After total occlusion occurs clinically, however, the performance at the phacoemulsification tip is similar to that of the peristaltic pump. The vacuum level at the tip rises to the preset level of the internal pump while the flow rate drops to zero. When occlusion is relieved, the vacuum at the tip once again drops nearly to zero. The stored potential energy in the system is translated into the clinical phenomenon of surge, just as in a peristaltic system. After the surge phenomenon, the flow rate stabilizes at the level determined by the internal vacuum of the Venturi pump.

Next, the personal ID programming saves up to 30 sets of profiles or personalized parameters. Each set or profile can contain various settings for each of the following parameters:

- Foot pedal—cautery preset
- Low vacuum/high vacuum phaco mode presets
- Low vacuum/high vacuum I/A mode presets
- Vitrectomy mode presets—vacuum settings
- Pump/flow settings

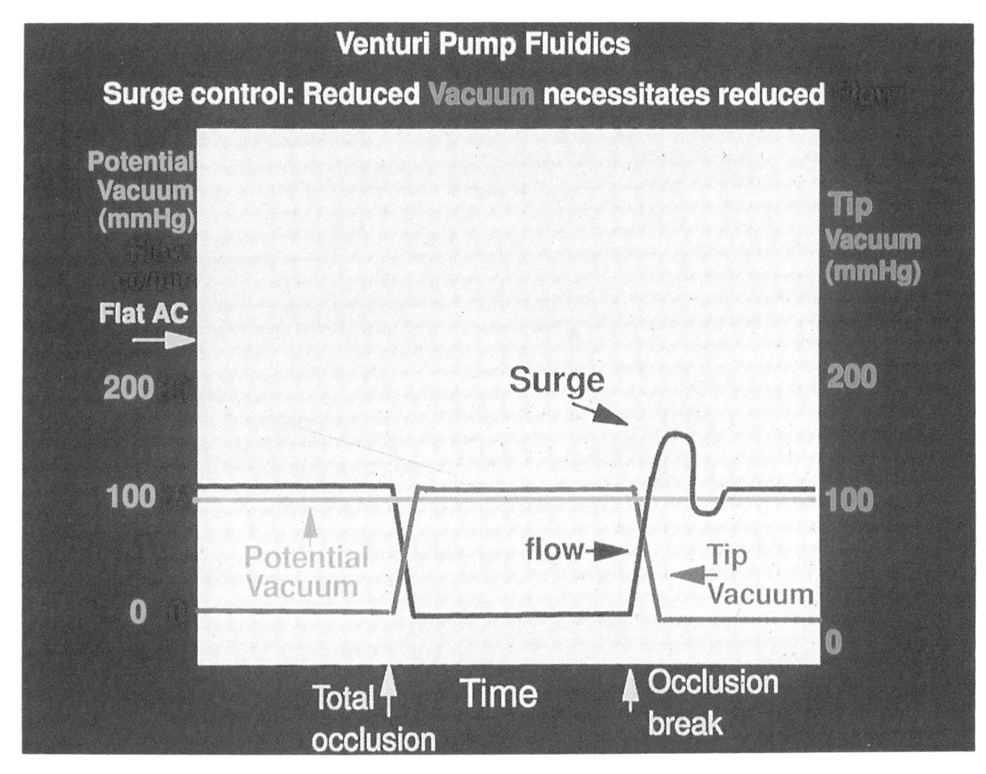

Figure 3-3F. To compensate for surge and to maintain the anterior chamber, typically both maximum potential vacuum and flow rate are reduced. Because of the intrinsic linkage of flow and vacuum in a Venturi or diaphragm pump system, reduction of the internal potential vacuum necessitates a reduced flow rate. By reducing both the flow and maximum vacuum, the surge level can be reduced below the level of flattening of the anterior chamber.

These features enable consistent parameters for the surgeon from case to case, as well as customization of the machine parameters according to surgeon preferences and surgical requirements.

Finally, the Control Center remote control enables adjustments of surgical parameters from the surgical field.

Fluidic control during irrigation/aspiration is at least as important as during phacoemulsification. In fact, studies have shown that more posterior capsules are ruptured during irrigation/aspiration than during phacoemulsification. Irrigation/aspiration is fully programmable, with a choice of linear flow or linear vacuum. Linear flow allows the surgeon to control the speed of attracting material to the I/A tip. Linear vacuum utilizes a preset flow rate but then controls the vacuum level in occlusion with the foot pedal. Linear vacuum seems familiar to users of traditional peristaltic systems, whereas linear flow gives some of the versatility typically associated with Venturi or diaphragmatic units. With experience, many peri-

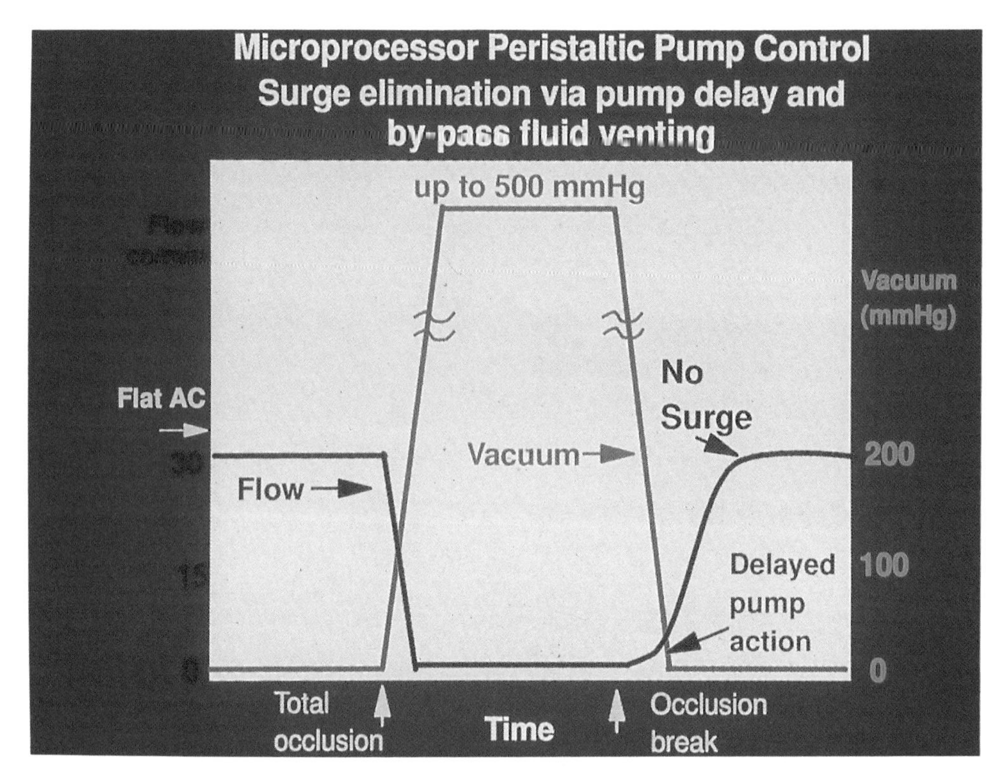

Figure 3-3G. New computer technology in the AMO Prestige unit offers enhanced control over the surge phenomenon. As a result, phacoemulsification can be performed at vacuum levels that were previously highly unsafe. As illustrated, a microprocessor peristaltic pump control system may allow vacuum levels to safely build up to 500 mmHg. After a break in the occlusion, the microprocessor delays the action of the pump by delaying its onset and speed of acceleration by microseconds. This is imperceptible to the surgeon. Combined with other steps such as reducing the compliance of the vacuum tubing, the phenomenon of surge is reduced to clinically tolerable levels, and high vacuum can be employed as a clinical tool without danger of collapse of the anterior chamber. Reproduced with permission from Steinert RF. *Cataract Surgery.* Philadelphia, Pa: WB Saunders; 1995.

staltic pump surgeons learn to appreciate the control of events that linear flow affords.

The unit also offers linear control of cautery. Because the amount of electrical cautery energy varies considerably depending upon surgical conditions as well as the electrical cord connections, linear control allows adequate cauterization without thermal injury and shrinkage of tissues.

Because of its intuitive, user-friendly design, operating room staff who are not frequent users of the device will nevertheless be able to help a surgeon experience a smooth and calm operative procedure. Adjustments are easily made during surgery to any of the key parameters through the remote control or the panel.

Personal Experience

My personal experience with the AMO Prestige Unit currently consists of over 500 procedures. My preferred technique combines the high vacuum capabilities of the Prestige Unit with the technique of Phaco Chop which was introduced by Dr. Kunihiro Nagahara. I utilize my Phaco Chopping "claw" instrument, manufactured by Rhein Medical (Tampa, Fla), in order to sequentially disassemble the nucleus into "bite-sized" pie-shaped wedges that are aspirated and sequentially emulsified in a controlled fashion, so that there is only one small fragment at any given time.

Phaco Chop can certainly be fruitfully employed with or without high vacuum; similarly, high vacuum is a very useful adjunct to any surgeon, whether or not Phaco Chop, quadrant divide and conquer, or other techniques are employed. It is my personal feeling that the high vacuum capabilities of the AMO Prestige Unit are particularly well suited to Phaco Chop, however.

The Phaco Chop maneuver allows the surgeon to create, in an exquisitely controlled fashion, fragments of nucleus that are appropriate for high vacuum phaco aspiration with minimal ultrasound power.

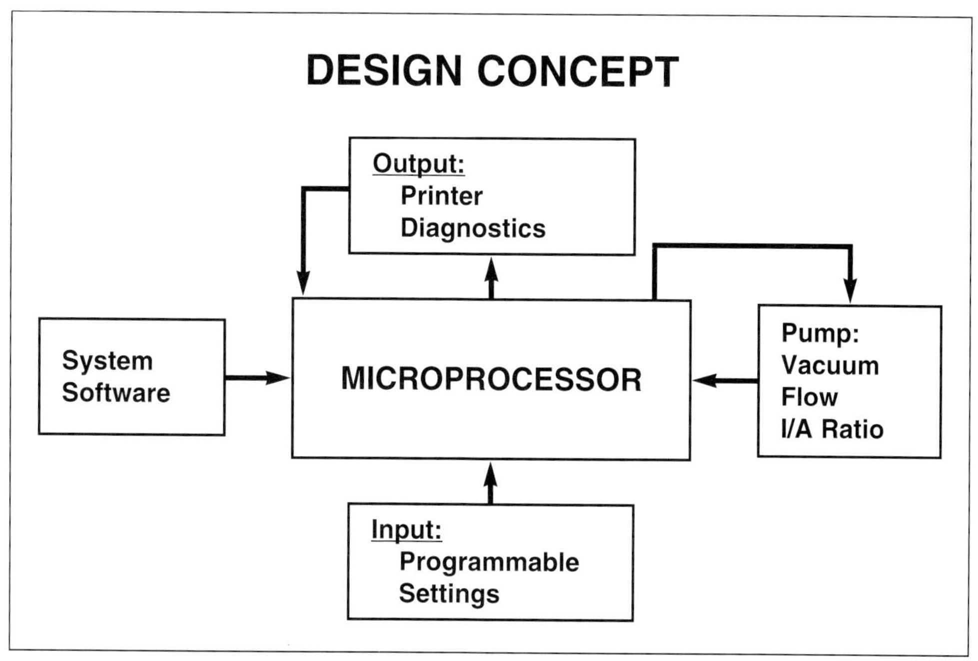

Figure 3-4. Block diagram illustrating the design concept and information flow of components of the AMO Prestige Unit.

The phacoemulsification unit engages the nucleus and high vacuum levels are allowed to build while the tip is in occlusion. The nucleus is drawn slightly toward the center, exposing the border of the nucleus and epinucleus. The chopper can then be safely introduced into this space, and a pie-shaped nuclear wedge is "chopped" with the second instrument. Ultrasonic energy can then directly aspirate the nuclear fragment, or a small burst of ultrasound energy will cause the wedge of nucleus to break down into an aspiratable fragment. The nucleus is removed in a safe and controlled fashion with the minimum amount of ultrasonic energy.

Preoperatively, I grade the expected nuclear hardness of each cataract, based on the appearance of the lens, principally consisting of nuclear coloration, combined with the patient's age. Nuclear hardness is graded on a scale of 1 through 4. I then use one of four programmed memory settings corresponding to my estimation of the nuclear hardness preoperatively. If I find that the nucleus behaves differently during surgery, the parameters can then be adjusted appropriately. The typical memory settings that I employ for the four degrees of nuclear hardness are given in Table 3-7.

Because of the exquisite microprocessor control of the AMO Prestige Unit, I can maximize the vacuum energy that is appropriate for a given level of nuclear hardness, without having to worry about post-occlusion surge or having to adjust the aspiration rate. The microprocessor will automatically decrease the aspiration rate to match the vacuum level and degree of occlusion. The anterior chamber is therefore stable, and I can employ high vacuum power to maximally "phacoaspirate" and minimally "phacoemulsify."

Table 3-1. Sources of Energy for Nuclear Disassembly

♦ Ultrasound
♦ Second instrument
♦ Vacuum
♦ Irrigation flow
♦ Laser

Table 3-2. Reduction of Ultrasonic Energy Through High Vacuum

♦ Improvement in ultrasonic coupling
♦ Direct fragmentation of the nucleus
♦ Aspiration of larger fragments

Table 3-3. Design Goals of the AMO Prestige Phacoemulsification Unit

♦ Reduction of ultrasonic energy through optimization of fluid dynamics
♦ Maximize flexibility of responsiveness, flow capacity, and range of safe vacuum
♦ Fully programmable to customize device parameters

Table 3-4. High Ultrasonic Energy Surgery

♦ Advantages	Visual feedback: nuclear decomposition
	Audible feedback
	Faster overall surgery
♦ Limitations	Less control
	More potential for complications
	More phaco energy → more heat

Table 3-5. Low Ultrasonic Energy Surgery

♦ Advantages	Slower → more control
	Less phaco energy → less heat
	Less heat → minimize trauma to wound, cornea, iris
♦ Limitations	Longer overall surgery
	Less effective with dense cataracts
	Less adaptable within a procedure

Table 3-6. Description of a "Powerful" System

- ♦ Attracts nucleus, good "followability"
- ♦ Holds nucleus, regardless of size or technique
- ♦ Emulsifies nucleus smoothly, regardless of cataract density
- ♦ Evacuates nucleus while maintaining stable chamber

Table 3-7. Dr. Steinert's Settings for AMO Prestige Unit

	AMO Prestige Nuclear Hardness			
	1+	2+	3+	4+
Phaco Power	40%	60%	70%	80%
Pulse Setting	Continuous	Continuous	Continuous or 16 PPS	Continuous or 16 PPS
Sculpting (low memory)				
Maximum Vacuum (mmHg)	70	80	100	100
Flow (cc/min)	26	26	26	26
Linear (flow/vacuum)	Flow	Flow	Flow	Flow
IV Height (cm)	60	60	60	60
Chopping (high memory)				
Maximum Vacuum (mmHg)	100	200	300	400
Flow (cc/min)	24	26	26	26
Linear (flow/vacuum)	Flow	Flow	Flow	Flow
IV Height (cm)	77	77	89	89
Epinucleus				
Maximum Vacuum (mmHg)	100	140-160	140-180	140-200
Flow (cc/min)	26	26	26	26
Linear (flow/vacuum)	Flow	Flow	Flow	Flow
IV Height (cm)	77	77	77	77
I/A				
High (cortex, viscoelastic)				
Maximum Vacuum (mmHg)	500	500	500	500
Flow (cc/min)	28	28	28	28
Linear (flow/vacuum)	Flow	Flow	Flow	Flow
IV Height (cm)	71	71	71	71
Low (vacuum capsule)				
Maximum Vacuum (mmHg)	50	50	50	50
Flow (cc/min)	10	10	10	10
Linear (flow/vacuum)	Vac	Vac	Vac	Vac
IV Height (cm)	31	31	31	31

Vitrectomy settings

Maximum Vacuum: 125 mmHg; Flow: 10 cc/min; Cut Rate: 10 cuts per second; IV Height: 31 mm.

Vitreous alone: pedal 2 steps; vitreous plus cortex: 3 steps.

Pedal span: 2-8-5.

I/A=irrigation/aspiration; IV=intravenous.

Chapter 4

Phacoemulsification with the Chiron Vision Phacotron Gold

John D. Hunkeler, MD

Introduction

The Phacotron Gold (Figure 4-1) is a phacoemulsification machine manufactured by Chiron Vision of Claremont, California. In addition to phacoemulsification, the Phacotron Gold also enables surgeons to comfortably perform extracapsular surgery, irrigation and aspiration procedures, and anterior vitrectomy. I will review the many key components of this machine and will then look at what the machine has to offer during surgery.

Key Components of the Phacotron Gold

Phacoemulsification with the Phacotron Gold is enhanced by a number of features, including the following:

- Binary fluidics pump
- Lightweight Magnum-Mini phaco handpiece
- Smooth ultrasonics

- Easy front panel access and control
- Remote diagnostic system
- Unique AVPC (Automated Vent Port Connection) tubing connection
- Easy-to-use expert keys memory system for retaining surgical parameters
- Cost-efficient usage

Binary Fluidics Pump

The system has a peristaltic pump that builds vacuum upon occlusion and then vents to air rather than fluid. It mimics the responsiveness of Venturi and diaphragmatic machines, while at the same time providing the control of the peristaltic technology. The Phacotron Gold uses stepper-motor technology, which allows the pump to turn on and off instantaneously. The microprocessor that controls the motor spins it rapidly based upon the aspiration rate. With aspiration rates in the 26 to 30 cc range the Phacotron Gold's rise time to 100 mmHg is comparable to that of a Venturi or diaphragmatic system.

A Lightweight Magnum-Mini Phaco Handpiece

The ergonomically designed Magnum-Mini is 1 inch shorter than Chiron Vision's previous handpieces. As a result, it offers the surgeon more clearance during phacoemulsification and facilitates temporal approaches used for clear-corneal procedures. Because there are no external irrigation lines, the handpiece can also be rotated much like a pencil, offering more flexibility in surgery. In addition, its all-titanium construction combined with its small size makes it one of the most lightweight handpieces available. For the doctor this lightweight ergonomic design means less hand fatigue during the phacoemulsification procedure.

This small lightweight design proves particularly advantageous when operating in the steep meridian, especially temporally, in the eye opposite that of the dominant surgical hand, which for a right-handed surgeon this would mean the patient's left eye and for a left-handed surgeon would mean the patient's right eye. Since the handpiece is small, it can make holding the instrument directly in front of the surgeon easier.

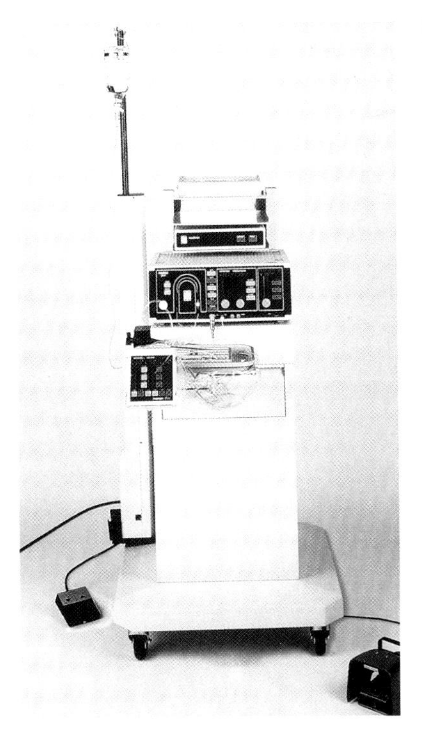

Figure 4-1. Phacotron Gold.

Smooth Ultrasonics

A 40-kHz handpiece with Autosense tuning of the ultrasonic driver replaces the traditional presurgical tuning cycle. The ultrasonic driver is constantly adjusting to the changing conditions within the eye resulting in more consistent, controlled power to the tip during phacoemulsification. This allows for more efficient cutting, enabling the surgeon to cut through and remove material from the nucleus without unnecessarily generating additional energy within the eye not needed for the procedure.

The Phacotron Gold is continually retuning itself as it goes from harder to softer nuclear material, to help avoid inadvertently cutting through the capsule. With the Phacotron's autotuning feature, cutting remains consistent throughout the surgery.

Also, the fact that the surgeon is using power more efficiently allows for cooler temperatures at the incisional site. When doing clear-corneal phacoemulsification this results in less trauma from thermal effects that may occur at the wound.

Easy Front Panel Access and Control

An easy-to-read front panel allows the surgeon and staff to quickly see the parameters that are currently programmed into the machine. They also get a real-time readout on exactly what is occurring, with a numeric display and accompanying bar graph that shows the energy that is actually being delivered. The easy-to-reach panel can also be quickly reprogrammed at any time with the touch of a single key.

Remote Diagnostic System

The remote diagnostic system, called CIA (Computer Interrogator Application), uses a telephone modem hook-up to the Phacotron Gold that allows the company's service department to be on-line with the customer and the machine at the same time. This enables representatives to efficiently diagnosis any difficulties with the Phacotron and determine whether the problem is the result of operator or machine error.

For example, while individuals may be convinced that they have loaded the machine's tubing properly, many times they have not. The CIA system quickly identifies the problem. In cases where a machine component is in fact broken, the on-line diagnostics will allow service representatives to ensure that the needed part is on hand before the arrival of the customer's machine so that it can be returned to the customer within a day, thereby reducing surgical downtime.

Unique AVPC (Automated Vent Port Connection) Tubing Connection

The Phacotron's tubing set features an AVPC (Automated Vent Port Connection). This unique feature ensures that the tubing is properly aligned to the pump-head before surgery begins and also minimizes any problems with fluidics that may otherwise occur during the procedure as a result of set-up errors. With prior technology, many surgeons did not notice leaks in the tubing system or take note of aspiration problems until they had already begun the procedure and were unable to build any type of vacuum. The AVPC allows the system's self-diagnostics to check in advance and aid the staff to ensure that this does not happen.

Easy-to-Use Expert Keys Memory System

A memory key system allows surgeons to store their individual operating parameters. This helps to ensure a repeatable, consistent set-up of the machine before each procedure and enables assistants to quickly reconfigure variations in flow, vacuum, and power for each individual surgeon.

Cost-Efficient Usage

The Phacotron Gold uses an automated vent-port connection on both the disposable and reusable tubing systems, helping to maintain lower usage cost. Also, the ease with which the equipment can be set up between cases translates into reduced turnover time.

Phacoemulsification with the Phacotron Gold

I have refined my technique in surgery to the point that not a single movement is wasted. I am in tune with all the motions in surgery and am constantly striving to reduce cycle time by optimizing steps, eliminating unnecessary motion, and seeking efficiency and consistency. Within this framework, the Phacotron Gold affords a straightforward solution, paired with good visual results and predictable refractive outcomes for the vast majority of patients.

The ease with which the equipment can be set up between cases is the first point. This translates into reduced turnover time and the ability to do more procedures. In refining incision procedure, I have found the machine's lightweight Magnum-Mini phaco handpiece to be particularly useful.

In addition to traditional incisions, I have moved to a clear-corneal temporal approach. The lightweight Magnum-Mini phaco handpiece allows easy and comfortable maneuverability, regardless of the location of the incision.

Using the Phacotron Gold for phacoemulsification, I perform the standard four-quadrant nucleus cracking technique. Two essential elements for nucleus removal include phaco power responsive to various tissue density and on-demand vacuum control. I prefer to let the built-in technology auto adjust the power level through various tissue densities, while focusing on the patient and the procedure. Also, no time or effort is wasted while waiting for vacuum or venting. The system is responsive to the foot switch, thus I do not have to compensate for delays (Table 4-1).

Given the shorter phacoemulsification time, another time-saving feature is the use of the continuous irrigation or infusion. When constantly on and off the foot switch, the chamber remains deep for the next phaco pass.

Another essential aspect of time saving is the reliability. Prior to surgery, the machine does not need to be readjusted between cases by the doctor or by the scrub nurse.

Summary

The Phacotron Gold is a dependable, versatile machine that allows the surgeon to perform phacoemulsification without making many adjustments during the procedure itself or when going from patient to patient.

The lightweight Magnum-Mini phaco handpiece offers the surgeon comfort and flexibility, and the system's peristaltic pump, with stepper-motor technology, allows for vacuum-on-demand, comparable to that offered by Venturi and diaphragmatic technology.

The Phacotron Gold is a straightforward machine that works in a consistent fashion.

Table 4-1. Chiron Vision Phacotron Gold with 30 Degree Radial Tip

	Memory Key—Dr. Hunkeler			
	U/S	**I/A**	**Capsule Polish**	**Viscoelastic Removal**
Irrigation	Continuous	Foot switch	Foot switch	Foot switch
Power	50%			
Aspiration	22/cc	40/cc	10/cc	40/cc
Vacuum	85 mmHg	500 mmHg	20 mmHg	500 mmHg
Mode	Linear	L-Vac	Panel	L-Vac

Chapter 5

THE OMS DIPLOMAX IN ENDOLENTICULAR PHACOEMULSIFICATION

Samuel Masket, MD
Richard Thorlakson, MD

Introduction

Current methods for successful lens nucleus removal depend heavily upon the performance characteristics of the phacoemulsification unit. Significant advances in fluidics, ultrasonics, and software development have enabled the machinery to perform reliably and to match the demanding needs of advanced phacoemulsification surgical styles. Most current surgical methods require disassembly of the nucleus within the confines of the lens capsular bag. Generally, several stages are performed in sequence. The first step involves sculpting or the formation of a groove or grooves, followed by some form of nuclear fracture (cracking, chopping, etc), and removal of the divided portions of the nucleus. Next, the epinucleus is aspirated with or without lens cortex. Each stage of the surgery requires specific setting of machine parameters for maximum performance. Additionally, given the "density" of any cataract, it may be necessary to alter the cutting and aspiration parameters for each of the emulsification steps.

My style of choice for phacoemulsification is based upon a divide and conquer method with hydrodelination and quadrisection of most nuclei in the fashion of crack and flip phaco; some lenses (5%) are too soft for fracture methods but aspirate well with occasional bursts of emulsification, and others (5%) are sufficiently hard to require additional fracturing.[1] I tend to prefer the use of an aspiration system for the quadrants based primarily upon high flow rate rather than ultrahigh levels of vacuum, since, in my view, the latter may be threatening to the posterior capsule, given the possibility of chamber collapse after fluidic occlusion break.

Therefore, it is desirable for emulsification equipment to be flexible and allow for easy change of parameters during surgery. The OMS Diplomax phacoemulsifier offers a series of unique hardware and software innovations that give the surgeon intraoperative flexibility, control, and safety. These additional features are not only innovative, they are functional and helpful for any phaco technique. The ultimate benefit to the OMS Diplomax is that it adjusts to fit any technique; one need not adjust his or her technique to fit the machine. Following a presentation of these innovations, I will discuss how I utilize them in my preferred style of phacoemulsification.

The Basics

The OMS Diplomax (Figure 5-1) evolved from the OMS Diplomate phacoemulsifier and shares all of its basic features. It is microprocessor driven; provides phaco, I/A, vitrectomy, and diathermy capabilities; and utilizes an air-vented peristaltic pump to generate precisely controlled aspiration.

There has been much discussion in the literature concerning the preferred type of pump to use on a phaco machine. In my experience, the air-vented peristaltic pump is the most controlled and forgiving, especially during the phaco portion of the procedure. It avoids the excessive tissue grabbing associated with a Venturi pump and a fluid-vented peristaltic pump. The "grabbiness" of these kinds of pumps results from the extremely fast vacuum rise at the phaco tip following occlusion. With the air-vented peristaltic pump there is time to react to the events occurring at the phaco tip so that one stays in control, even when using fast aspiration rates. The air-vented system also allows for exquisite low vacuum stability when performing "zero vacuum" phaco and when vacuuming the posterior capsule in CapVac mode with the I/A handpiece.

Eight different user-defined programs can be identified on the Diplomax screen by surgeons' names, nucleus density (soft, medium, hard), and age of patient (under 40, 40 to 50, 50 to 60, etc). All parameters in all modes can be independently set for each program. It is not necessary to rely on ancillary staff to adjust the parameters to the surgeon's preferences. Multiple Modulation Phacoemulsification (MMP) is available within each of the eight user-defined programs. This allows for immediate access to three distinct sets of phaco parameters with the touch of a single button.

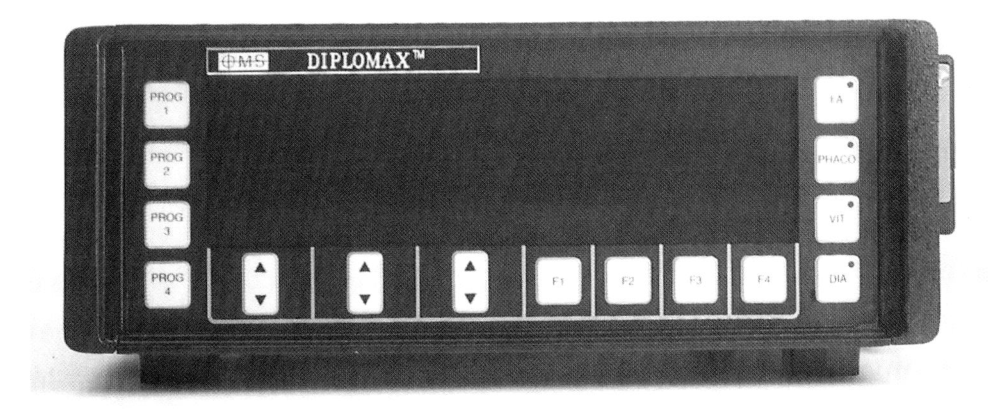

Figure 5-1. The OMS Diplomax.

Sculpting can be done with zero vacuum and continuous power in Phaco 1, quadrant removal can be done with high vacuum and pulsed power in Phaco 2, and epinucleus can be removed with a fast aspiration rate and low power in Phaco 3. This makes nucleus removal much more efficient and much safer. The surgeon has significantly more control over the procedure. Logical and precise changes to all surgical parameters can be made during the procedure. Preset and actual values for each parameter are displayed simultaneously on the Diplomax screen in an easily understood format using definitive values (cc/min, mmHg, percent power). The following is a list of additional basic features found on the Diplomax:

User Interface Features

- Full function total remote control
- On-screen step-by-step set-up instructions
- Color-coded tubing set-up
- Automated prime cycle
- Automated tuning cycle with continuous autotuning
- Error prevention software

- On-screen troubleshooting
- Choice of disposable or reusable tubing
- Programmable IV pole
- Articulated arm and tray
- Adjustable height machine stand
- Programmable foot pedal detent positions

Intraoperative Features

- Instantaneous vacuum venting
- Foot pedal-activated gravity reflux
- Handpiece power-off feature
- Pulsed/continuous ultrasound power
- Linear/panel ultrasound power
- Linear/panel aspiration
- Audio feedback for vacuum, aspiration rate, occlusion, and ultrasound
- I/A with ultrasound mode
- Side-Vit vitrectomy mode
- CapVac mode

Postoperative Features

- Automated end-of-case purge cycle
- Automated end-of-day cleaning cycle
- Ultrasound timer with Equivalent Phaco Time (EPT)
- Upgradable by changing computer chip

Therefore, the Diplomax incorporates all the basic features typically found on the most advanced phacoemulsifiers. It is from this point forward that the Diplomax departs from the traditional and offers the following innovations.

Programmable Vacuum Rise Time

How fast the vacuum rises in phaco mode, **after** occlusion of the phaco tip occurs, can be customized for each surgeon's preference for each stage of the procedure. There is very little, if any, vacuum at the end of a phaco tip until it becomes occluded, regardless of which type of pump is being used. Significant vacuum is only produced following occlusion of the tip. With a peristaltic pump, the rate of vacuum rise following tip occlusion is directly proportional to the aspiration rate (or pump speed.) A high aspiration rate will produce a fast vacuum rise. A low aspiration rate will produce a slow vacuum rise. With the Diplomax, it is possible to program an Occluded Aspiration Rate that is independent of the Preset Aspiration Rate set for the unoccluded state. Thus, one could set a low aspiration rate setting with a slow or fast vacuum rise, or a high aspiration rate setting with a slow or fast vacuum rise.

By programming a very slow vacuum rise with a low aspiration rate, the need for zero vacuum sculpting can be eliminated. Since the vacuum will rise very slowly, the surgeon has time to react to any undesired occlusion by releasing the foot pedal before any undesired material is aspirated. This allows some degree of available vacuum to extend the sculpted trough out to the periphery in a very controlled manner.

By programming a fast vacuum rise with a low aspiration rate, removal of the nuclear quadrants will be more controlled and efficient. With a low aspiration rate, a quadrant can be picked up without unintentionally attracting the surrounding epinucleus to the phaco tip. Once occlusion occurs, the vacuum will rise quickly to maintain a grip on the quadrant to hold onto it as it is pulled into the center of the chamber for emulsification.

By programming a slow vacuum rise with a high aspiration rate, removal of the epinucleus will be more controlled and efficient. With a high aspiration rate, the epinuclear shell will be attracted out to the phaco tip held in the center of the chamber. The phaco tip will not have to be extended out into the periphery of the bag to grasp the epinucleus. Then, once the epinucleus has come out to occlude the phaco tip, a slow vacuum rise will allow for a gradual rise in vacuum to aspirate the epinucleus into the phaco tip. The slow vacuum rise gives you sufficient time to release the foot pedal if iris or capsule are inadvertently attracted to the phaco tip. Removal of the entire epinuclear bowl will be very controlled and efficient, particularly with a moderate vacuum limit in combination with pulsed phaco to encourage removal of the epinucleus when the moderate vacuum alone is not sufficient. Using moderate vacuum instead of high vacuum for removal of epinucleus will eliminate the problem of the vacuum biting off a small piece of epinucleus with each occlusion. The entire bowl can be held onto and manipulated with moderate vacuum and then aspirated with the assistance of pulsed phaco as necessary.

Automated Vacuum Venting

A concern often voiced about an air-vented peristaltic pump is the phenomenon known as "vacuum surge" following the sudden release of an occlusion of the phaco tip. This concern is addressed by the Diplomax with its in-line vacuum sensor which senses when an occlusion breaks. At that instant the Diplomax automatically vents the vacuum in the line to atmosphere to prevent the surge. This provides remarkably stable anterior chambers at significantly higher vacuum levels, while maintaining the low vacuum benefits of an air-vented peristaltic pump.

Double Infusion Pinch Valve

There are two separate infusion pinch valves on the Diplomax. The surgeon has the choice of using a standard one bottle set-up or a two bottle set-up with the two bottles of BSS hung at different heights to give different infusion pressures and flows. The Diplomax can be programmed to use the low bottle when low aspiration rates and low vacuums are being used and to use the high bottle when high aspiration rates and/or high vacuums are being used. The change in infusion pressure will be immediate, without having to wait for the programmable electric IV pole to change the bottle height.

Autopulse Phaco

If Autopulse Phaco is turned on, at high phaco powers the phaco handpiece will run in continuous power mode. As the foot pedal is relaxed into lower powers, the phaco handpiece will automatically change to pulsed power. This is particularly useful when sculpting the nucleus. When sculpting the hard central core of the nucleus at higher powers, the handpiece will be running in the continuous mode for smooth and efficient cutting. When extending the trough out to the periphery (at which point low powers are used), the handpiece will automatically change to pulse mode, giving more exquisite control of cutting than would using low power alone. There will be less likelihood of inadvertently cutting through the epinuclear rim and catching capsule.

Burst Mode Phaco

Burst Mode Phaco yields bursts of ultrasound power when the foot pedal is in position 3. Each burst will be at the preset power level (non-linear). There are three programmable choices as to the length of each burst: 40, 60, or 80 milliseconds. At foot pedal position 3-**Minimum**, the bursts will be 2 1/2 seconds apart. As the foot pedal is depressed further into position 3, the bursts will get closer and closer together until, at foot pedal position 3-**Maximum**, the bursts will blend together and the power will become continuous (at the preset power level.) This is useful in quadrant management for techniques that emphasize vacuum to remove the quadrant assisted by intermittent bursts of ultrasound power. The surgeon can control the frequency of the power bursts without coming off and on the foot pedal.

Occlusion Mode Phaco

The power modulation of the phaco handpiece (continuous, pulse, autopulse, burst, power off) can be programmed to automatically change when the phaco tip is occluded versus unoccluded, in any combination desired. This has a variety of applications.

During sculpting, the Diplomax could be programmed to automatically change from continuous power to pulsed power when the tip occludes. This gives immediate feedback regarding any undesired occlusion, either at the phaco tip or even a kink somewhere along the tubing. Extending the trough at 6 o'clock will be done with the added control of pulse mode without having to change settings. Furthermore, this will decrease the likelihood of an inexperienced phaco surgeon getting a corneal burn from embedding the phaco tip into the nucleus and running high continuous power with no aspiration flow to cool the handpiece. Having the Diplomax change to the "power off" mode when the tip occludes would make sculpting even more controlled for the beginning surgeon.

A possible combination to control nuclear quadrants would be to program the Diplomax to automatically change from pulsed power to burst mode power when the tip occludes. The pulsed power is used to "lollipop" into the quadrant to obtain occlusion. The quadrant is then pulled to the middle of the chamber and the handpiece automatically changes to burst mode power to assist the vacuum in the removal of the quadrant.

The epinucleus could be managed by programming the Diplomax to automatically change from a long pulse mode to a short pulse mode when the phaco tip occludes. The long pulses will help initiate occlusion and then the short pulses will allow for very controlled removal of the epinuclear bowl, particularly in combination with the slow vacuum rise capabilities described earlier.

Foot Pedal Remote Control

With the Diplomax, one can switch the phaco memory setting (Phaco 1, Phaco 2, or Phaco 3) with the foot pedal. It is not necessary to ask an assistant to change the settings on the face of the machine, or on the handheld remote control, when changing from sculpting to quadrant removal to epinuclear tumbling. This facilitates the use of the different memory settings for the different stages of the procedure, thus making the procedure more controlled and efficient for the surgeon.

Personal Application

The beauty of the Diplomax is that one only needs to use the features that benefit the individual surgeon. One simply programs the desired features. Each of the eight surgeons that can be programmed into the Diplomax can individually select each of the functions that they desire.

Surgical Methods

The Diplomax parameters I use for each phase of surgery for a typical cataract are noted in Table 5-1 and Figures 5-2 through 5-4, and surgery is planned as follows. Following capsulorhexis, hydrodissection (often with attempted cortical cleaving), and hydrodelineation, the emulsification handpiece is introduced with the infusion at low bottle height (approximately 30 cm). Low bottle height prevents sudden deepening of the anterior chamber, thus avoiding "ciliary body stretch" which may

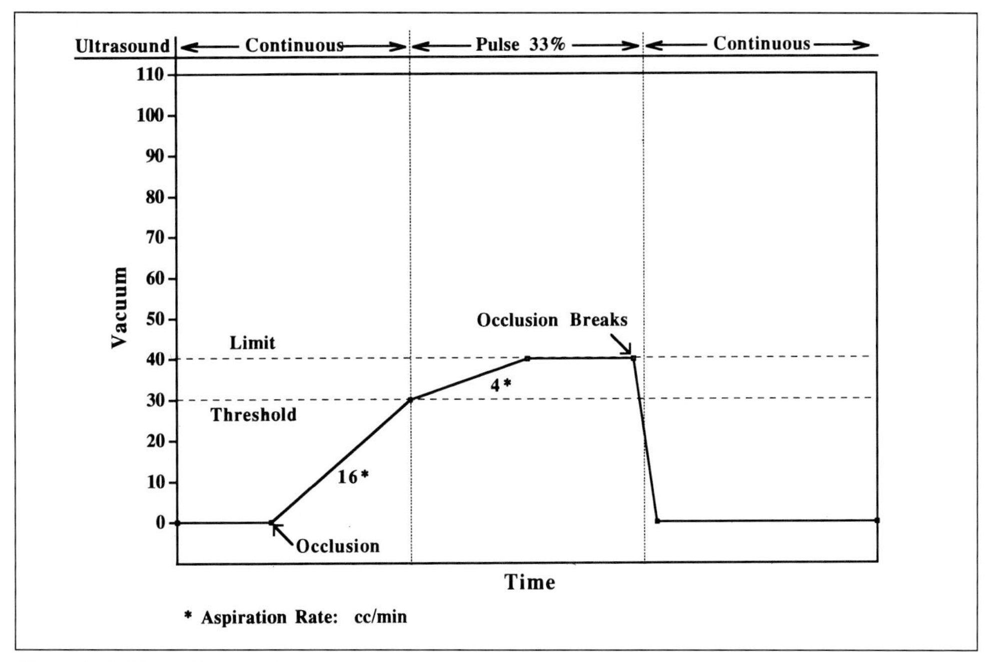

Figure 5-2. Phaco 1: sculpting.

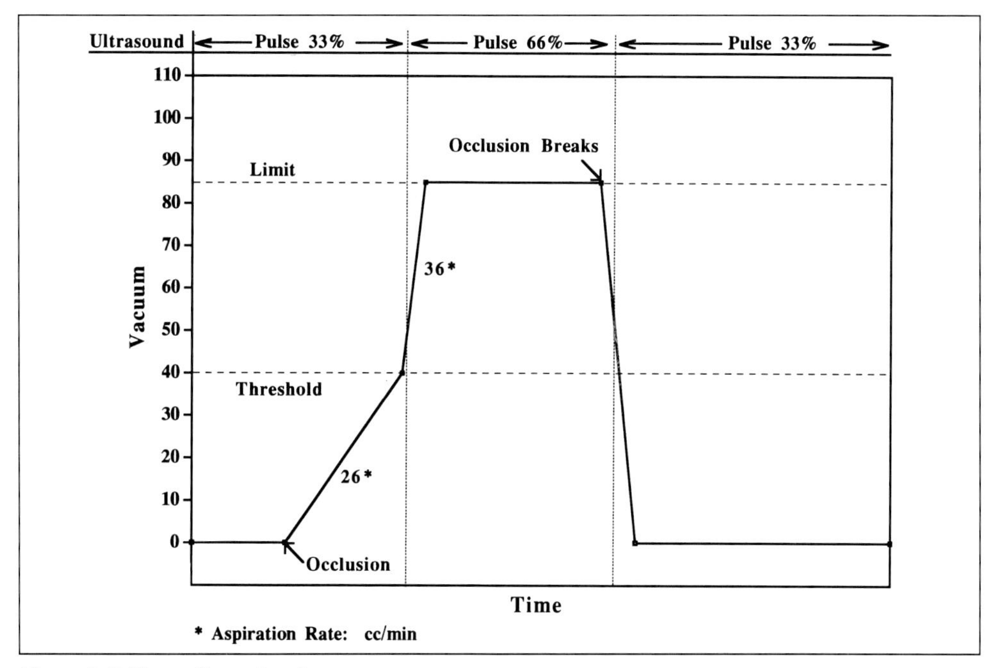

Figure 5-3. Phaco 2: quadrants.

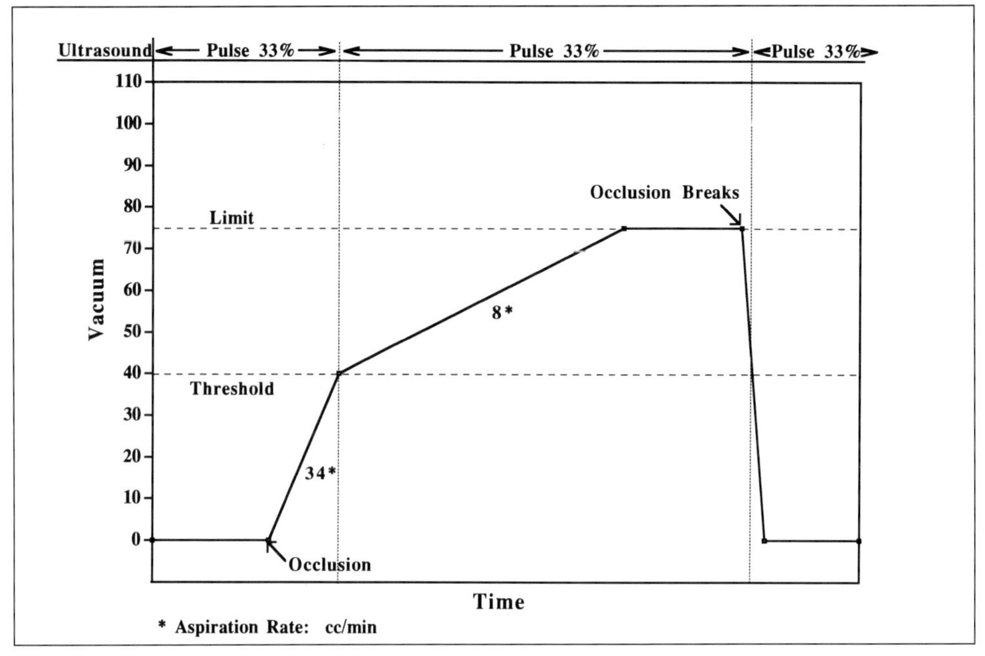

Figure 5-4. Phaco 3: epinucleus.

induce pain for those patients having surgery under topical anesthesia. Although not part of the Diplomax system, I use an ergonomically designed and angled phacoemulsification tip (Masket Ergo Tip) which provides for ease of groove sculpting and cuts more efficiently than a traditional straight tip (Figure 5-5). Generally, I opt for the fluidic behavior of a 30° angled tip, but I will employ a 45° tip for extremely hard lenses, given the fact that higher tip angles cut more proficiently. During sculpting I use a spatulated collar button instrument in my second hand to hold, turn, and manipulate the nucleus. Very low vacuum setting (so-called zero vacuum phaco) is associated with a slow turnover of debris from the anterior chamber, limiting the surgeon's view. The purported safety of low vacuum rates is obviated with the unique software capabilities of the Diplomax, which allow for changes in the fluidics and emulsification modes as occlusion of the tip is sensed by the microprocessor. As noted in Table 5-1, during groove sculpting, when the tip is unoccluded, the aspiration rate is preset at 16 cc/min and vacuum may reach 40 mmHg. However, as I sculpt deeper into the groove and reach more peripherally, the tip may occlude. At that moment, the phacoemulsification mode changes from continuous surgeon control to pulsed phaco, indicating to me that the tip is occluded. While I may use this "early warning device" to change the sculpting stroke, the fluidics change auto-

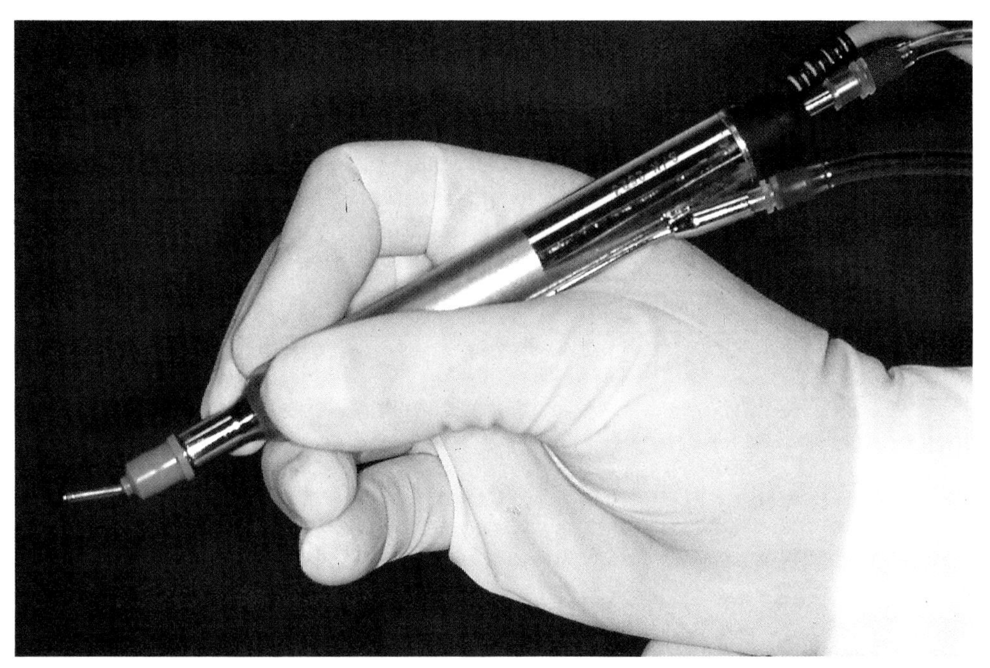

Figure 5-5. The Diplomax phaco handpiece with angled phaco tip (Masket Ergo Tip) provides a physically comfortable, ergonomically sound tool for surgery.

matically to reduce aspiration to only 4 cc/min, once a vacuum threshold of 30 mmHg is reached. This automatic change in rise time offers me great safety when sculpting the primary groove either deeply or peripherally; it reduces surgery time while affording good visibility. I rotate the nucleus 180° to complete the primary groove and bisect the nucleus using the phaco tip and second instrument. Next, a 90° rotation brings one portion of the hemisected nucleus into position to create the secondary grooves which are cut in a different manner than the primary groove. The secondary grooves need only be long enough to accommodate the left (second) hand instrument. Sculpting is performed by taking advantage of the safety net provided by the software since I often impale the tip and create a short tunnel. The fact that the phaco mode switches to pulse when the tip is occluded prevents tip heating. Cracking is performed by holding the nucleus with the phaco tip in a lollipop maneuver and using the second instrument to break the heminucleus into two parts, an inside-out form of nuclear "chopping." Lollipopping may be facilitated by using burst mode, wherein the occluded tip will stop after a series of short bursts. The remaining heminucleus is sectioned in similar fashion and the quadrants are ready for removal.

The nuclear fragments are removed by working within the confines of the epinuclear shell in most cases. However, when working with very firm lenses I tend to bring the quadrants away from the capsule to the deepest part of the chamber since the epinucleus may be very thin or non-existent, offering little protection to the peripheral or posterior capsule. I shift the machine from Phaco 1 to Phaco 2 with the foot pedal, eliminating the need and waiting time for the assistant or circulator. The infusion line is elevated (programmable) to accommodate for the increased flow and vacuum used during quadrant removal. The second instrument elevates the apex of the quadrant away from the posterior capsule while the phaco tip is embedded into the thickest portion of the nuclear chunk. Burst mode phaco enables the quadrant to be impaled and easily controlled; final removal is performed within the epinuclear shell or in the deepest portion of the chamber. Quadrant removal is greatly facilitated by the software modifications of the Diplomax. In my Phaco 2 settings, after the nuclear piece is mobilized and is lollipopped, the aspiration flow rate will increase from a preset 26 cc/min to 36 cc/min after occlusion is sensed. Consequently, the vacuum limit (which I set at 85 mmHg for most cases) will be reached more rapidly since the rise time is proportional to the aspiration rate. During quadrant removal, pulse mode phaco is employed. The pulse rate may be programmed according to the surgical plan. I use a shorter pulse (33%) prior to occlusion in order to prevent pushing the nuclear fragment away from the tip. However, once occlusion has occurred, the fragment is held well by the vacuum and the pulse length increases to 66% in order to efficiently aspirate the nuclear piece.

Epinucleus removal is performed in Phaco 3 position, again obtained by a simple movement of the foot switch, avoiding the need for the assistant or circulator to change machine parameters. The thickness of the remaining epinucleus varies with the size of the true nucleus and the zone of hydrodelineation. A very thick (or firm) epinucleus may require trimming on the top of the bowl in order to allow for easy flipping in the later stages of aspiration. The fluidic parameters that I choose allow for increased flow until tip occlusion occurs, after which the flow is reduced so that the bowl will be held but not fractured by the pull (vacuum) of the machine. Otherwise, pieces of the epinucleus may be inadvertently broken free, which is less desirable than being aspirated as a total mass. This avoids the need to have the tip reach into the fornices of the capsular bag. I use the purchase of the phaco tip to hold firmly on the epinuclear bowl while I use the second instrument to flip the shell by sweeping the superior portion of the remnant inferiorly as described originally by Howard Fine.[2] Once the epinucleus (with or without cortex) has been freed from the capsular fornices, aspiration is completed with occasional bursts of pulsed phaco, as needed, to keep the tissue moving along the phaco tip.

Cortical Aspiration

Occasionally, perhaps in 25% of cases, it is not necessary to remove cortex as a separate step, since cortical cleaving hydrodissection allows cortex to be aspirated with the epinucleus. However, it has been my experience that cortical cleaving may leave small wispy strands of cortex that are difficult to aspirate since they do not fill the port. As a result, vacuum cannot build up to clear the remaining fine cortical material. For that reason, I believe that it might be more efficacious, albeit slower, to remove cortex following epinuclear aspiration.

Nevertheless, the initial hydrodissection can aid eventual cortical clean-up. I prefer to hydrodissect toward the main incision (temporally) by way of the side paracentesis in order to facilitate subincisional cortex removal during the later stages of surgery. Generally, I complete cortical clean-up prior to lens implantation, since it is possible, although very rare, that cortex may become trapped under the lens or the capsular bag may be damaged in removing residual cortex. In case of the latter, the prior placement of a plate haptic lens would necessitate its removal. Should cortex be difficult to remove, however, it is wise to perform additional hydrodissection, viscodissection, or remove residual cortex following lens implantation. In routine cases I use a preset vacuum level of 500 mmHg and a flow rate of 18 cc/min. I employ surgeon control of aspiration rate.

Conclusion

Phacoemulsification continues to evolve as an exquisite art, combining manual dexterity of the surgeon with engineering genius and foresight. Improvements in machine capabilities allow similar results for each case type, so that the competent surgeon will have parallel positive experiences and successful results for virtually all cases. The unique software and hardware modifications afforded me by the Diplomax have reduced the challenges and increased the reproducibility of endolenticular phacoemulsification.

Table 5-1. Dr. Masket's OMS Diplomax Settings

	Phaco 1: Sculpting		Phaco 2: Quadrants		Phaco 3: Epinucleus		I/A
	unoccluded	occluded	unoccluded	occluded	unoccluded	occluded	
Aspiration Rate	16	4	26	36	34	8	18
Vacuum Level	(Limit) 40	(Threshold) 30	(Limit) 85	(Threshold) 40	(Limit) 75	(Threshold) 40	500
Power Level	60		60		40		
Power Mode	Continuous	Pulse 33%	Pulse 33%	Pulse 66%	Pulse 33%	Pulse 33%	Linear Aspiration ON

References

1. Fine IH, Maloney WF, Dillman DM. Crack and flip phacoemulsification. *J Cataract Refract Surg.* 1993;19(6):797-802.
2. Fine IH. The chip and flip phacoemulsification technique. *J Cataract Refract Surg.* 1991;17(3):366-371.

Chapter 6

Storz Premiere/MicroSeal System Description

Richard J. Mackool, MD

The Storz Premiere/MicroSeal System (Figure 6-1) is available as an anterior or an anterior/posterior microsurgical system capable of providing the following modes:

- Irrigation
- Irrigation/aspiration
- Phacoemulsification and phacofragmentation
- Vitrectomy
- Endoillumination
- Bipolar coagulation
- Intraocular pressure control

User Interface

The console is microprocessor controlled, electro-pneumatic, and contains a preprogrammable logic system which permits storage of individual surgeons' procedure parameters. The parameters which I currently recommend for various phases of phacoemulsification and for lens cortex removal are displayed in Table 6-1. All primary functions and self-diagnostic features are under the control of dedicated microprocessors. A soft-touch screen display is readily sterile covered to permit the scrub nurse control of all functions, and provides the operator with essential instructions, menus, and feedback concerning operation and functions. A handheld remote control is also available. The pneumatic and electronic circuitry are modular, implemented with circuit boards in a VME (VERSAmodule Europe) bus configuration for ease in servicing. The phacoemulsification/fragmentation mode is available for both anterior and posterior segment procedures. Phacoemulsification power can be delivered at a fixed level determined by the console control, in linear fashion during which power is foot pedal controlled and aspiration level is determined by console control, and PhacoAspiration™ mode during which vacuum level is determined by foot pedal control and phacoemulsification power is applied at a fixed level at any time and at a level which is determined by the console control.

The screen display provides a number of features which allows system flexibility by use of "soft," programmable switches. When a mode is selected on the console, the mode will be displayed in inverse video. The intensity of modes that are

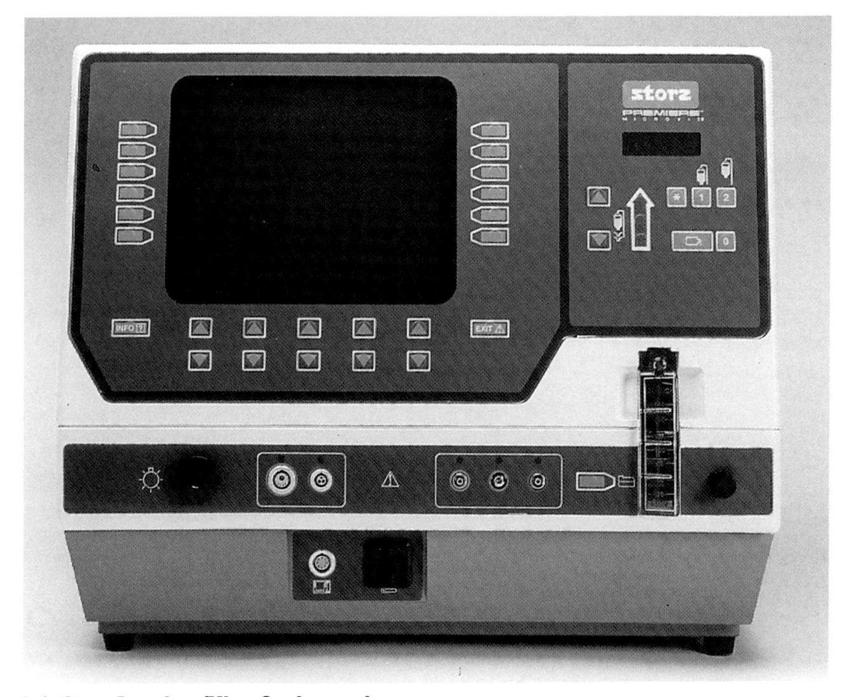

Figure 6-1. Storz Premiere/MicroSeal console.

temporarily unavailable will appear dimmed. The screen displays are arranged in a logical manner to assist operation of the system. A primary screen allows selection of anterior surgery, posterior surgery (anterior/posterior systems only), or utility functions. Secondary screens allow selection of the functions required for the surgical procedure or configuration of the instrument for a particular surgeon or purpose.

Ultrasonic Handpiece/Electronics

The MicroSeal ultrasonic handpiece utilizes a piezo-electric crystal, and operates at a frequency of 27 kHz. The system uses a resonant frequency sensor to analyze voltage, current, and power output. A patented servo mechanism then maintains power during phacoemulsification through the use of a closed-loop control.

The patented design of the MicroSeal tip utilizes dual infusion sleeves which surround the titanium ultrasonic needle (Figure 6-2). The outer silicone sleeve is manufactured with parameters which permit it to deform to the shape of an incision

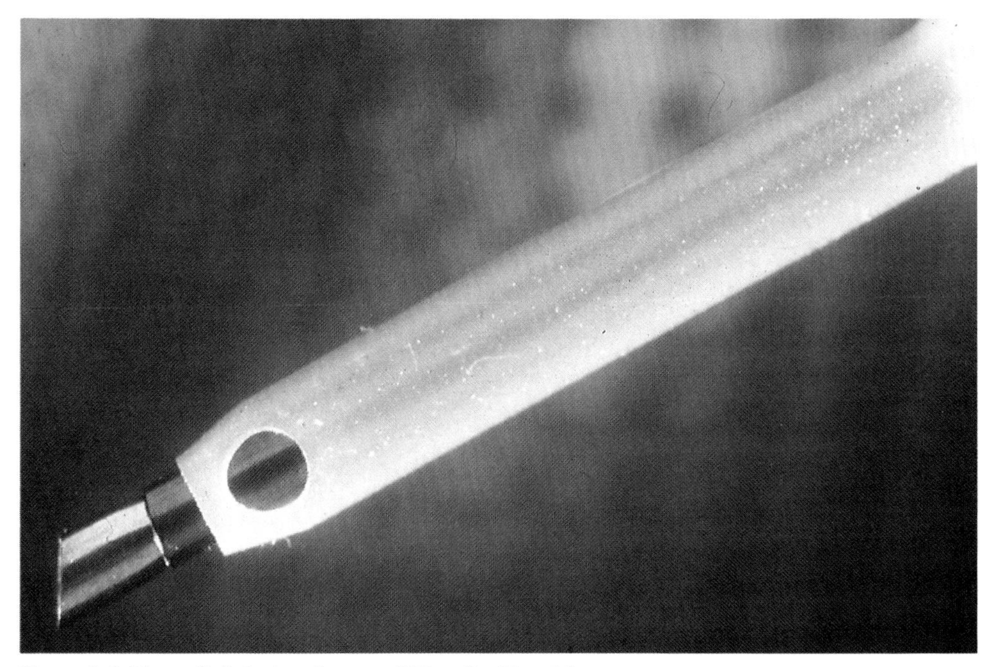

Figure 6-2. Phaco tip/infusion sleeves of MicroSeal handpiece.

of 2.2 to 2.5 mm, thus sealing the incision and preventing the incision from leaking. An inner rigid sleeve is present between the silicone sleeve and the ultrasonic needle. This sleeve does not permit the silicone sleeve to be compressed against the vibrating ultrasonic needle by the incision, and therefore acts to prevent friction, heat generation, and incision burn during phacoemulsification (Figures 6-3 and 6-4).

The vitrectomy handpiece operates with a guillotine cutting mechanism and is adjustable from 30 to 750 cuts per minute (Figure 6-5).

The Vacuum Rise Time (time interval required to achieve maximum preset vacuum level) is programmable and may be varied from 1.5 to 6 seconds. The extremely rapid response of the pneumatic circuit permits venting from maximum vacuum to 0 mmHg in less than 250 milliseconds (1/4 second). The console and handpiece can be prepared for use and calibrated in less than 1 minute.

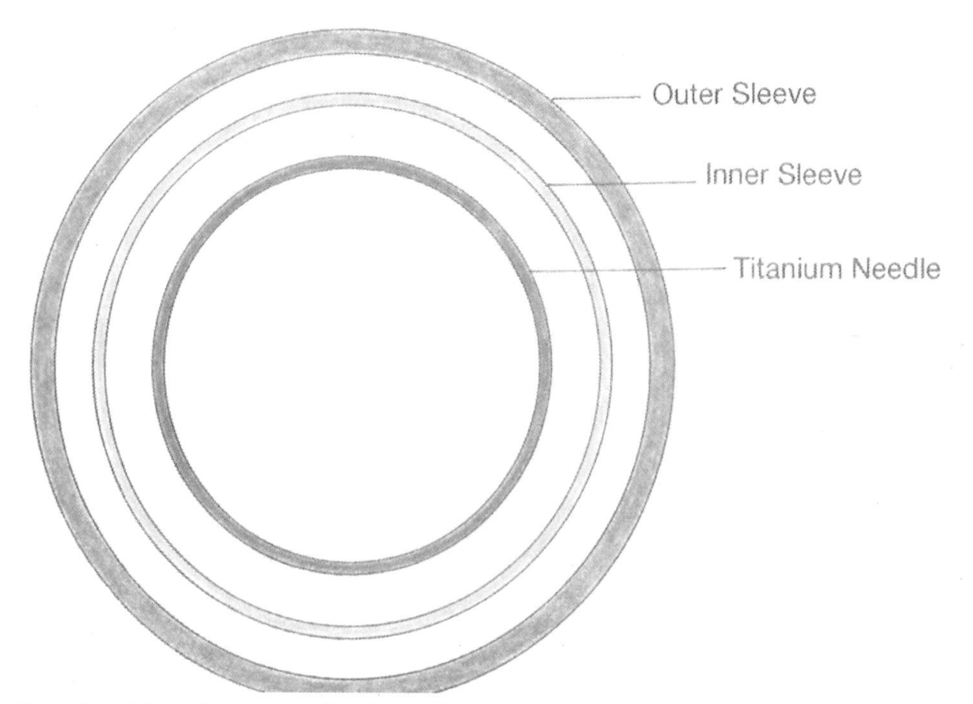

Figure 6-3. Schematic cross section through the tip of the MicroSeal handpiece. The central titanium needle is surrounded by a rigid sleeve, which is surrounded by a flexible silicone sleeve.

Fluidics

Fluidics refers to the behavior of fluid as it moves into, within, and leaves the eye. In order to discuss fluidics during phacoemulsification with the Premiere/MicroSeal system, a few simple definitions are required.

Flow. The rate at which fluid **enters** the eye from the infusion bottle and **exits** through any means, including the phaco tip, the phaco incision, or the side-port incision. I often refer to the cumulative amount of fluid that passes through the eye during a procedure as the "total fluid flow."

Aspiration Flow Rate. This is the rate of fluid leaving the eye **through the phaco tip** at any moment during surgery. The terms "aspiration" and "aspiration level" are confusing, and should not be used. Confusion stems from the fact that they are sometimes used to refer to aspiration flow rate, and at other times they are used to refer to vacuum level.

Vacuum. Vacuum is used to describe a negative pressure, ie, a pressure that is lower than the atmospheric pressure. In a Venturi system, vacuum is created by the

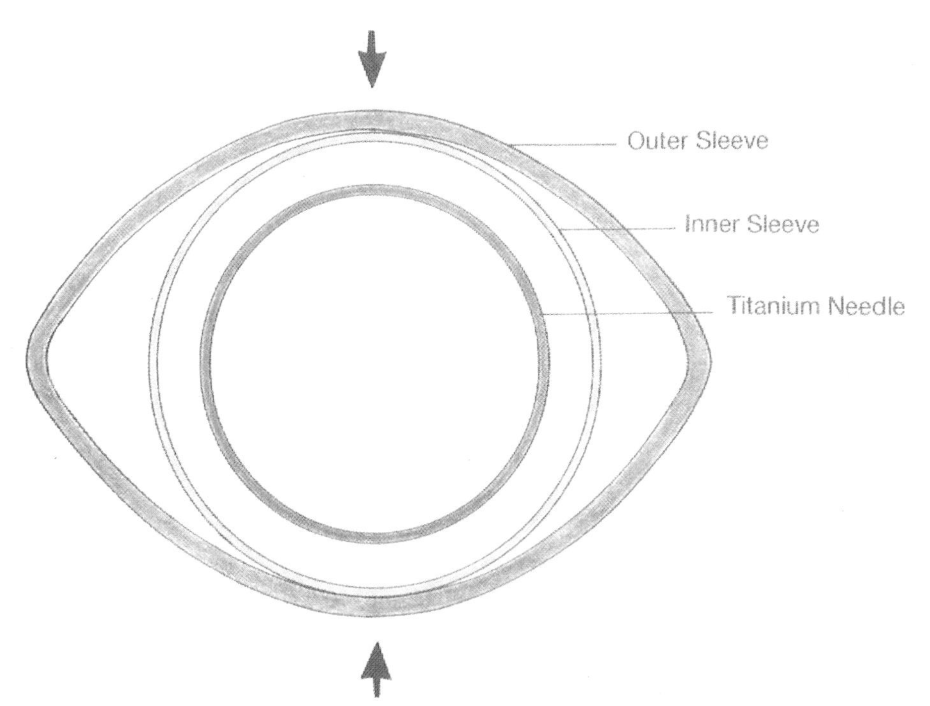

Figure 6-4. When inserted through a 2.2 to 2.5 mm incision, the flexible outer sleeve deforms to the elliptical shape of the incision, preventing incision leakage.

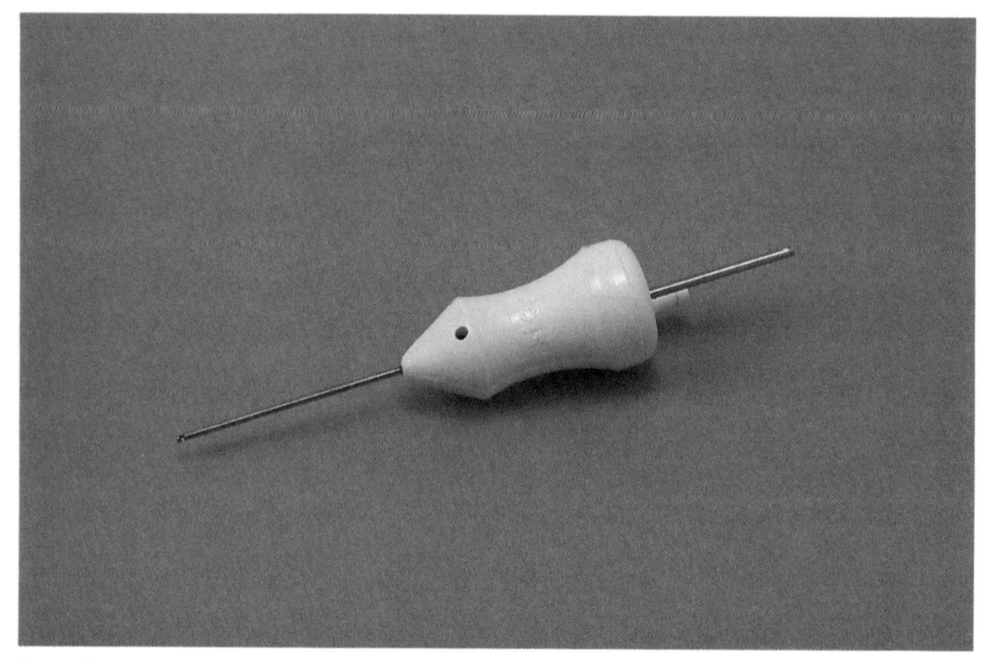

Figure 6-5. Twenty gauge vitrectomy probe (guillotine).

flow of compressed air or nitrogen through an orifice. This flow creates a vacuum in the cassette/aspiration line (Figure 6-6). The vacuum thus created controls the rate at which fluid leaves the eye. Therefore, the vacuum pressure directly determines the aspiration flow rate in a Venturi system.

Prior to the development of the MicroSeal system, leakage of fluid from the phaco incision during the procedure was constantly present during both the phacoemulsification and irrigation/aspiration portions of the surgery (Figure 6-7). The rate of this leakage is measurable, and varies between 15 and 40 cc/min when a standard, silicone-sleeved handpiece is inserted through a 3.0-mm incision. This remarkably high rate of flow through the incision results in more fluid passing through the incision and into the collection bag, at the side of the patient's head, than fluid flowing through a phaco handpiece. This situation persisted because inherent limitations of both flexible silicone and rigid (metallic or teflon) infusion sleeves do not permit them to be used in a manner which would prevent this leakage. With regard to silicone sleeves, an incision which is snug enough to prohibit leakage of fluid around the sleeve may promote an incision burn due to compression of the soft, flexible sleeve against the vibrating titanium needle, and subsequent production of heat by friction. If attempts are made to insert a rigid-sleeved instrument through a snug,

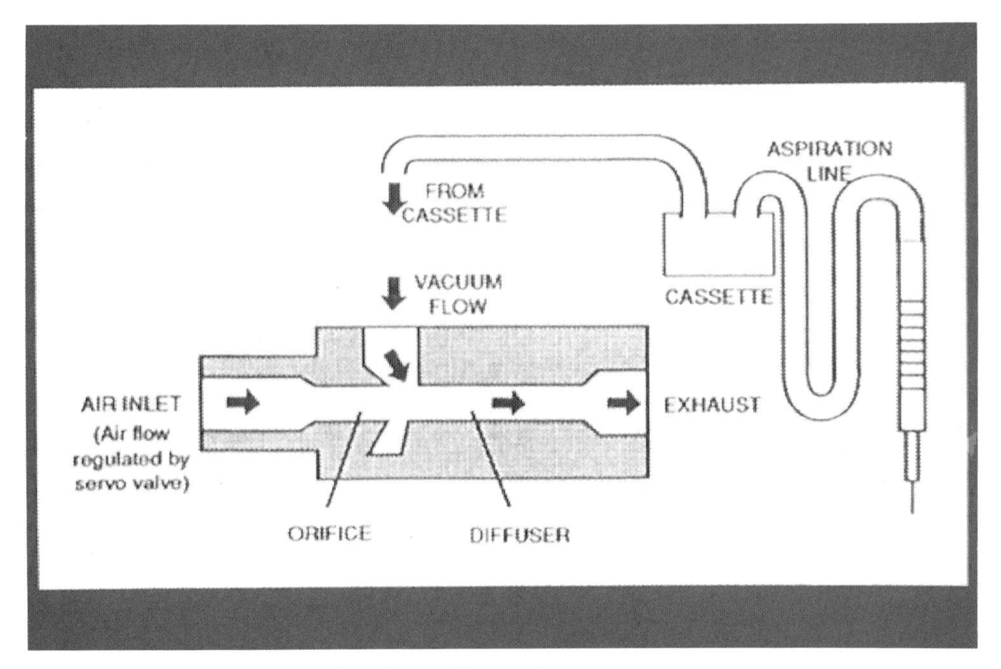

Figure 6-6. Schematic diagram of the Venturi flow system.

water-tight incision, undesirable corneal striae are created, and these greatly hinder visualization during the procedure. In addition, there is significant restriction of free movement of the instrument in a longitudinal direction during the operation. These effects are caused by the extremely tight fit which results from the deformation of the linear incision into the round configuration of the rigid sleeve. Therefore, the elimination of incision leakage by the use of a round, rigid sleeve has not been practical.

Fluid leakage from the incision during phacoemulsification and irrigation/aspiration is undesirable for several reasons. Excessive, turbulent flow through the anterior chamber is damaging to the corneal endothelium, and may cause increased postoperative inflammation as the iris is also traumatized by the rapid, turbulent movement of fluid. Perhaps more importantly, wide variations in intraocular pressure result from the incision leakage, creating fluctuations in anterior and posterior chamber volume, posterior capsule "trampolining," and variability in pupillary dilation (iris "flutter"). The position of iris and lens capsule are therefore very unstable, and chamber depth is much less than that which is consistently obtained when incision leakage is prevented (Figures 6-8 and 6-9).

Other problems created by incision leakage include decreased visualization, as

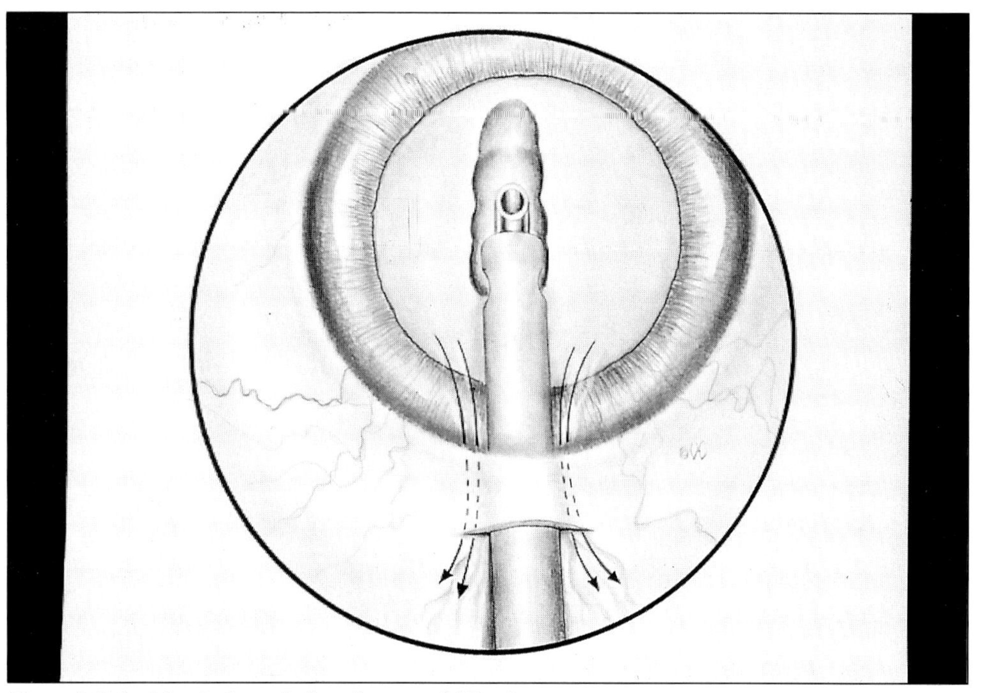

Figure 6-7. Incision leakage during phacoemulsification.

corneal striae are more readily induced when manipulations are performed in a soft eye. Followability of the nucleus is also severely reduced, as intraocular pressure reduction results in loss of the desirable pressure differential across the port of the ultrasonic needle, and the flow of fluid toward the incision creates undesirable vector forces which tend to carry nuclear particles away from the port of the phaco instrument. This situation therefore requires the use of a greater aspiration flow rate and/or vacuum level in order to establish the needed pressure differential across the ultrasonic port (Figure 6-10). This in turn decreases the safety of the surgical procedure by increasing the risk of chamber shallowing.

When intraocular pressure is maintained, it is also much easier to maintain or even increase pupillary dilation during phacoemulsification. This is due to the fact that pupillary constriction is often caused by intraocular hypotension and/or iris trauma. Eliminating incision leakage raises intraocular pressure, and the subsequent increase in chamber depth makes it far less likely that the surgeon will repetitively contact the anterior surface of the iris with the undersurface of the phacoemulsfication instrument.

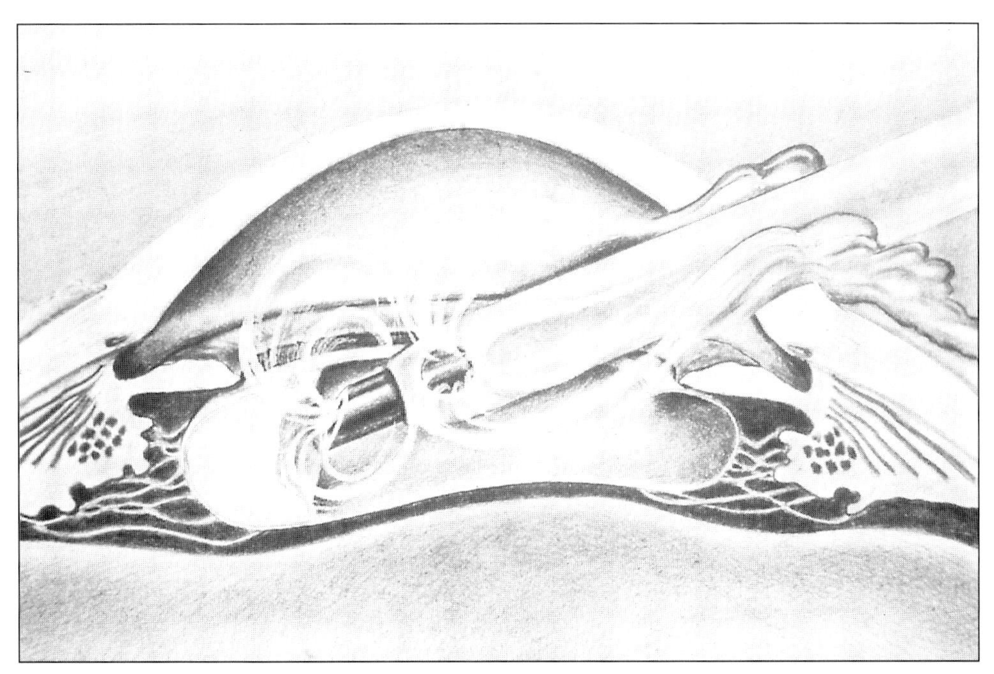

Figure 6-8. Intraocular turbulence and reduction of anterior and posterior chamber volume result from incision leakage.

Perhaps the above can be summarized with the following analogy. The advent of the large tennis racquet and oversized hitting surface of golf clubs have made the respective sports much easier to master. Can there be any doubt that increasing and maintaining the space in which phacoemulsification is performed will do anything less for the ability of surgeons to perform the procedure?

Phacoemulsification: Surgical Technique

The safe, efficient performance of phacoemulsification requires the appropriate use of technology and technique. With regard to the former, the instrument should be simple and thereby reliable, adequately sophisticated to provide precision, and these two requirements should be developed in such a way as to provide deep, stable anterior and posterior chambers; extremely rapid venting capacity; and efficient

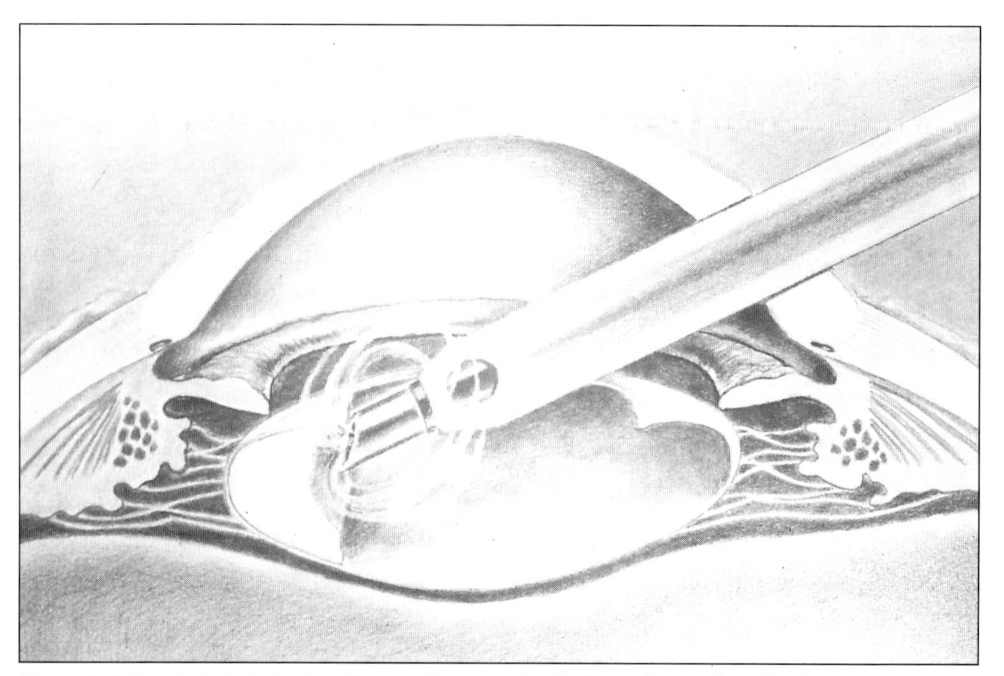

Figure 6-9. Non-turbulent, laminar flow and increased anterior and posterior chamber volume achieved by eliminating incision leakage.

application of ultrasonic energy. The previous sections have provided technical explanations for these achievements by the Storz Premiere/MicroSeal phacoemulsification instrument. This section deals with the manner in which this technology has permitted me to improve my technique and procedure.

Patient Selection for Phacoemulsification

The development of this instrument essentially permitted me to eliminate all prior contraindications to phacoemulsification, with only one exception: the cornea must be clear enough for me to see the instrument within the eye. Therefore, regardless of the preoperative endothelial cell count, chamber depth, pupil size, or even zonular status, I now perform phacoemulsification on every patient undergoing cataract extraction. This statement should not be taken to be a recommendation that the reader do the same. For example, the performance of phacoemulsification in instances of zonular dehiscence or lens subluxation should probably be restricted to those surgeons who are comfortable in removing lens fragments from the vitreous and/or surface of the retina by the pars plana approach. With this exception, however, I believe that the vast majority of surgeons will be able to perform phacoemulsification successfully in nearly every patient utilizing this technology. A discussion of the conditions which previously required extracapsular extraction, but for which I now routinely perform phacoemulsification with this technology, follows.

Preoperative Reduced Endothelial Cell Density

The tremendous reduction in total fluid flow through the eye during phacoemulsification with the Premiere/MicroSeal system has, in my experience, virtually eliminated all endothelial cell loss. This was demonstrated by the following study. Twenty consecutive patients underwent phacoemulsification with intraocular lens implantation utilizing the MicroSeal handpiece in January 1993. In January 1994, wide field endothelial cell photography was repeated by the same independent observer. In comparing the pre- and postoperative endothelial cell counts in these 20 patients, mean endothelial cell loss was 2.9%, and 40% of patients had no demonstrable cell loss. In addition to the findings of this study, I have operated on approximately 40 patients whose preoperative endothelial cell counts were so low as to be impossible to determine. These patients all had advanced corneal endothelial (Fuchs') dystrophy, yet had no preexistent corneal epithelial edema. An example of a preoperative endothelial cell photograph taken of one of these patients is shown in Figure 6-11. In every instance, the cornea has remained clear in these patients from the first postoperative day. The condition of the corneal endothelium, therefore, is no longer a factor in the decision to perform phacoemulsification on any patient with compromised endothelium.

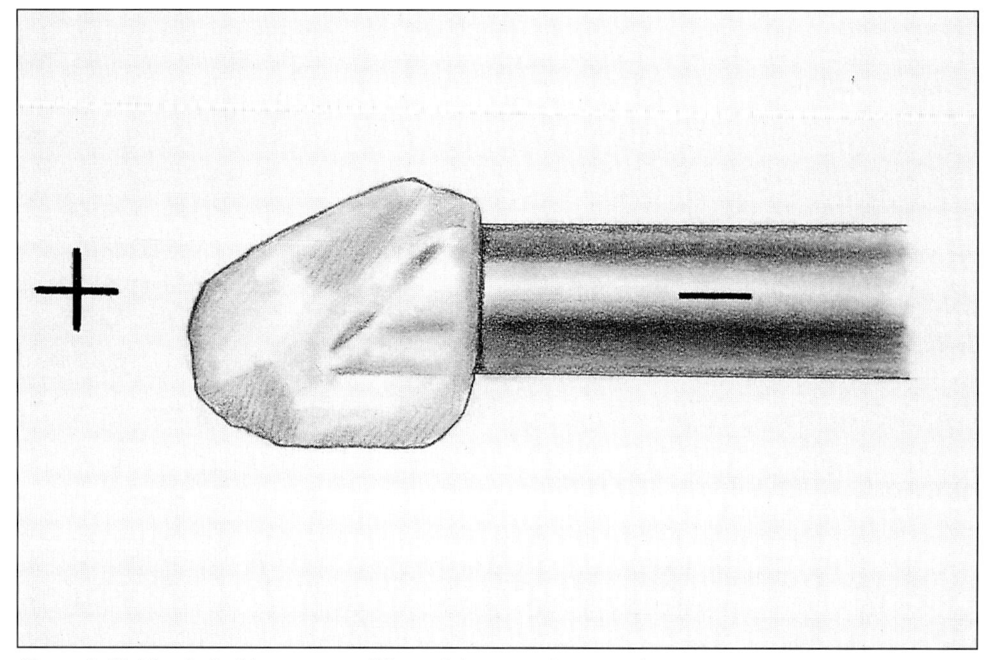

Figure 6-10. The desirable pressure differential across the part of an ultrasonic needle is created by increasing the IOP (+) and/or reducing the pressure (-) within the ultrasonic needle.

Preoperative Shallow Chamber

The Premiere/MicroSeal system eliminates incision leakage and increases intraocular pressure during phacoemulsification, and therefore creates a deeper chamber in every patient. Thus, even patients with preexisting shallow chambers nearly always maintain an adequate chamber depth during the procedure. Exceptions to this are rare but possible. I have had two patients whose chamber depth preoperatively was approximately 1.0 mm, and greater chamber depth could not be obtained by any surgical maneuvers. In order to achieve satisfactory anterior chamber volume in these patients, it was necessary for me to perform a limited pars plana vitrectomy, removing 1/2 to 1 cc of vitreous. Thereafter, viscoelastic injection into the anterior chamber did result in significant deepening and the procedure could be safely performed. Both of these patients demonstrated significant zonular laxity and porosity as evidenced by the fact that delivery of infusion fluid into the anterior chamber during pars plana vitrectomy did not result in significant chamber deepening. Such an event is absolute evidence of communication between the anterior and posterior segments, and this pathway is clearly through the lens zonule.

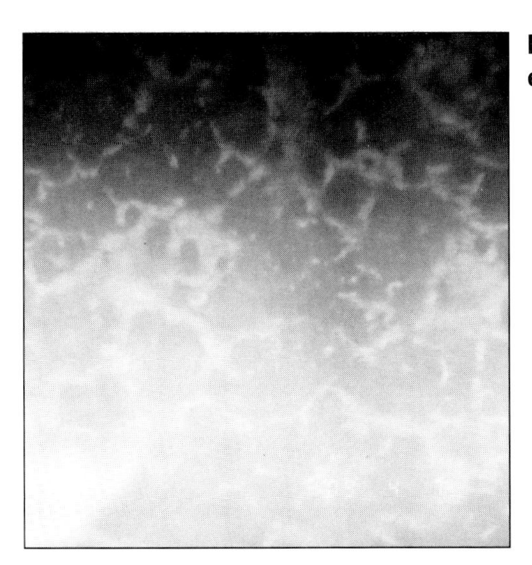

Figure 6-11. Extremely advanced corneal endothelial dystrophy.

However, pars plana vitrectomy, followed by injection of the anterior chamber with viscoelastic, was successful in creating a deep anterior chamber in each of these patients. As a final note, the development of an infusion misdirection syndrome might easily occur during phacoemulsification in such eyes, and careful observation for its development is required.

Incision Size

The incision size required for the MicroSeal handpiece is 2.2 to 2.5 mm, and I currently use a 2.4-mm keratome to create a clear-corneal or scleral-tunnel incision. As foldable lenses are successfully inserted through ever smaller incisions, this ability to perform phaco through the smallest possible opening becomes an obvious benefit.

Nuclear-Cortical Hydrodissection

In my experience, the increased anterior and posterior chamber volume and stability of IOP during phacoemulsification with the Premiere/MicroSeal system makes it unnecessary to intentionally separate nucleus from epinucleus prior to the performance of phacoemulsification. The purpose of this maneuver, ie, to leave the epinucleus as a capsular shield during phacoemulsification, is not required when incision leakage around the phaco tip is eliminated and intraoperative IOP is stabilized. It is therefore my practice to perform only capsular-cortical cleaving hydrodissection, and to remove the epinucleus simultaneously with the lens nucleus.

Nuclear Sculpting

Nuclear sculpting within a completely sealed chamber provides significant benefits as well as at least one interesting phenomenon. Regarding the latter, occasional episodes of "nuclear dust" formation within the anterior chamber are visible during periods of nuclear sculpting. This represents the dispersion of fine, particulate lens material into the chamber in the vicinity of the phaco tip. Since these particles do not wash out of the incision, they become visible to the surgeon as a gentle plume rising from the area of sculpting. Should this material result in decreased visualization, it may be quickly aspirated by momentarily withdrawing the phaco tip from the nucleus with which it is engaged.

Of far greater importance to the surgeon, however, is the extreme precision with which nuclear sculpting can be performed. The phaco tip can be advanced into the peripheral nucleus with masterful control, and without the fear of sudden rim breakthrough or subsequent aspiration of equatorial lens capsule. This permits the peripheral nuclear rim to be thinned to whatever extent is desired and/or necessary to achieve nuclear cracking. This is extremely important, as both relatively soft, elastic nuclei and very dense nuclei require severe thinning of the nuclear rim before they can be successfully cracked.

Lastly, the MicroSeal handpiece is extremely powerful, and is capable of achieving a stroke length of 3.75 mils (.00375 inches). Thus, a maximum power setting of only 30% is sufficient to easily remove the vast majority of nuclei. Extremely dense (red, black) nuclei may require a power setting as high as 50%.

Nuclear Segment Removal

The greatest advantage afforded by the closed system during this portion of the procedure results from the greatly expanded anterior segment volume. The latter permits the nuclear quadrants to be removed rapidly, at the level of the iris or in the posterior chamber, while a large distance between the nuclear segment and the corneal endothelium is maintained. Nuclear quadrants can be removed in the posterior chamber by elevating and attacking the apex of the quadrant, or the body of the quadrant can be impaled by the phaco tip, drawn into the center of the chamber, and removed. During the latter maneuver, it is not uncommon for the quadrant to tumble (Figure 6-12), but the presence of an extremely deep chamber guarantees that this event will be entirely innocuous. In addition, should the surgeon wish to attract the quadrant into the center of the chamber without impaling it, an aspiration pressure setting of 140 mmHg will create an aspiration flow rate which is sufficient to accomplish this.

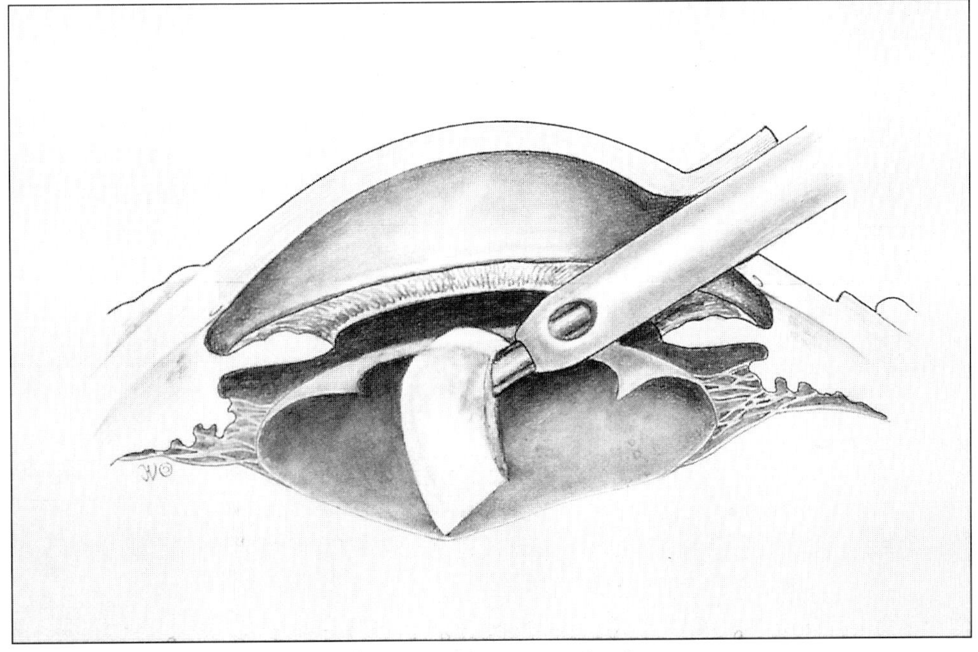

Figure 6-12. Tumbling of a nuclear quadrant within a deep chamber.

Nuclear Followability

Nuclear followability, ie, the ability to attract nuclear particles to the phaco tip and/or aspirate nucleus which is at the tip, is enhanced when operating in a sealed chamber. There are no competing vector forces created by fluid flow toward the incision, and the significantly greater intraocular pressure automatically creates an improved pressure differential across the ultrasonic port (difference between the pressure within the eye and the pressure within the phaco needle). Nuclear particles will not be carried toward the incision, but rather will remain in the vicinity of the ultrasonic tip where they are easily aspirated.

Phaco Chop

This very efficient means of nucleus segmentation is best performed while the nucleus is impaled by the ultrasonic tip, and is therefore stabilized within the posterior chamber (Figure 6-13). The ability to employ higher vacuum levels provides

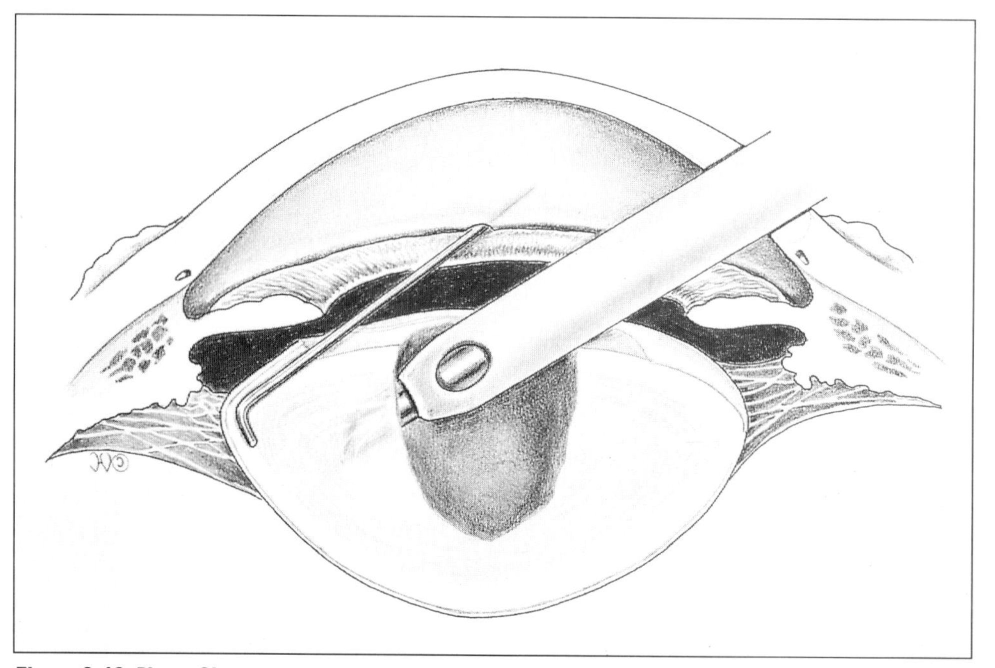

Figure 6-13. Phaco Chop.

the surgeon with a firmer "grip" upon the nucleus and an aspiration pressure of -160 mmHg can be used for this purpose. It is best to elevate the infusion bottle to 40 inches (distance between drip chamber and patient's eye level) when employing this vacuum level with the Venturi system.

Cortex Removal

The greatly expanded capsular sac, which is present when irrigation/aspiration is performed in a closed chamber, provides great benefits during cortex removal. A 90° angulated I/A tip can be used to remove cortex from all regions of the capsular fornix (Figure 6-14), and exchange of this handpiece for a straight I/A tip is therefore unnecessary.

There is a greatly reduced likelihood of accidental posterior capsule aspiration due to the presence of the deep, enlarged posterior chamber and concave, taut posterior capsule. Also, in those instances where accidental posterior capsule aspiration

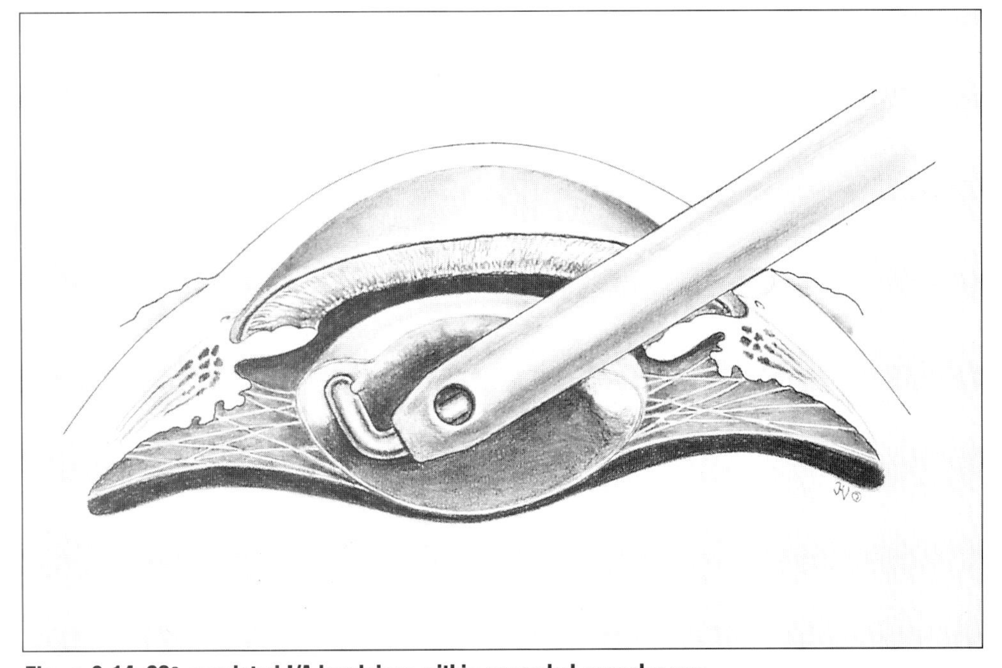

Figure 6-14. 90° angulated I/A handpiece within expanded capsular sac.

occurs, it is extremely unlikely that the posterior capsule will rupture as the rapid venting mechanism of the Venturi system provides immediate release of the capsule.

Incidence of Posterior Capsule Rupture/Vitreous Loss

Since I began using the Premiere/MicroSeal phacoemulsification system, my incidence of posterior capsule rupture/vitreous loss has declined dramatically. The frequency of this complication has fallen from 1.12% with the Premiere/standard handpiece, to 0.14% (1 per 738 operations) with the MicroSeal system. This retrospective study was conducted on anatomically normal eyes without preexistent zonular dialysis or dehiscence. The only downside here is that one may momentarily forget the appropriate response when confronted with this now rare complication. However, this is a small price to pay for the obvious benefit.

Perhaps the greatest benefit of this phacoemulsfication system is one which I only recognized in retrospect. Just as the anterior and posterior chambers are expanded during the procedure, so are the capacities of the surgeon. The increased confidence which results from working in a larger space is insidious but pervasive, and the vast majority of surgeons can be expected to perform more capably when their confidence level is elevated and their anxiety reduced.

Table 6-1. Storz Premiere/MicroSeal

	Sculpting	Quadrant Removal	Impale-Phaco Chop	Epinucleus Removal	
Power	30%*	30%*	30%*	30%*	I/A
Vacuum	30	100-120	160**		500
Mode	Continuous	Continuous	Continuous	Continuous or Pulse	I/A Mode

*Power settings of 40% to 50% are recommended when a very dense nucleus is present.

**Elevation of infusion bottle drip chamber to 40 inches above eye level is recommended.

Chapter 7

The Surgical Design Ocusystem II^ART

Harry B. Grabow, MD

Introduction

It was not only an honor for me to have been invited by Howard Fine to write this chapter, but a true privilege to have been able to review phaco history first-hand. In preparing the background for this manuscript, I requested technical information directly from the manufacturer, Surgical Design Corporation.[1]

The company's current president is William Banko, MD, the son and heir of the company's founder, Anton Banko, ME.[2] Anton, now deceased, was the former director of Cavitron's research group when he and Charles Kelman, MD, together, developed the first phacoemulsifier in the mid-1960s. Anton left his position with Cavitron and founded Surgical Design in 1967. In 1968, in collaboration with Charles Schepens, MD, and the Retina Foundation in Boston, he invented the first instrument for closed pars plana vitrectomy.

The original Ocusystem was introduced in 1980 with the collaboration of Buol Heslin, MD, and Richard Mackool, MD. It was the first single, computerized, intraocular microsurgical system to integrate phaco, irrigation/aspiration, and vitrectomy. Other advances in phaco technology can be attributed to Banko and contributors, such as pulse mode ultrasound (Jerre Freeman, MD, 1982) and the first 1 mm no-stitch endocapsular phaco (Steve Shearing, MD, 1984).

The next generation machine, the Ocusystem II^art, introduced in 1987, incorporated still further advances and now carried with it 26 phacoemulsification design patents and features. One of these innovative features was a transducer to sense sudden changes in intraocular pressure and vent to a closed fluid system, thereby uniquely suppressing vacuum surge and maintaining a stable anterior chamber. In 1991, Surgical Design introduced the Mini-Port Cobra Tip for more efficient delivery of ultrasonic energy. Subsequently, Adjustable Rise Time has recently been incorporated into the fluidics, allowing the surgeon to select a point along the vacuum curve at which the aspiration flow rate can be programmed to change automatically, faster or slower.

Surgical Design continues to remain a family-owned-and-operated, single-product company—the oldest in the business. As you can see by their ongoing, progressive, and pioneering spirit, they continue to be responsive to the industry.

Machine Components

The model currently manufactured by Surgical Design is the Ocusystem II^{art} (Figure 7-1). The main console has front panel controls with both LED digital visual display (Figure 7-2) as well as an audible vacuum level tone. The audible tone volume level is dialable and is continuous, increasing in pitch with increasing vacuum, converting to a beeping sound when the upper limit is reached.

A stand is available for the console with an attached instrument tray that is movable on a swing arm (Figure 7-3). Parameters may be adjusted and selected in unsterile fashion on the console or in sterile fashion by a wireless remote on the instrument tray (Figure 7-4). The main console also has an automated IV pole that holds two infusion bottles at two different heights (Figure 7-5). The lower bottle provides the fluid for routine irrigation, while the higher bottle provides the fluid for both reflux and venting.

Both reusable and disposable tubing are available for the Ocusystem II^{art}. The disposable tubing is clear polyvinyl chloride (PVC). The reusable tubing is translucent silicone and may be used between 50 to 100 times.[3] The tubing inside and outside diameters and wall rigidity are designed by intention to withstand vacuum pressures up to 500 mmHg without collapsing, while also providing the appropriate inflow for cooling, pressure, and volume maintenance.[4]

The machine is very user-friendly regarding set-up. Easy-to-follow guidelines are printed on the side of the console cabinet (Figure 7-6) for tubing connection. The

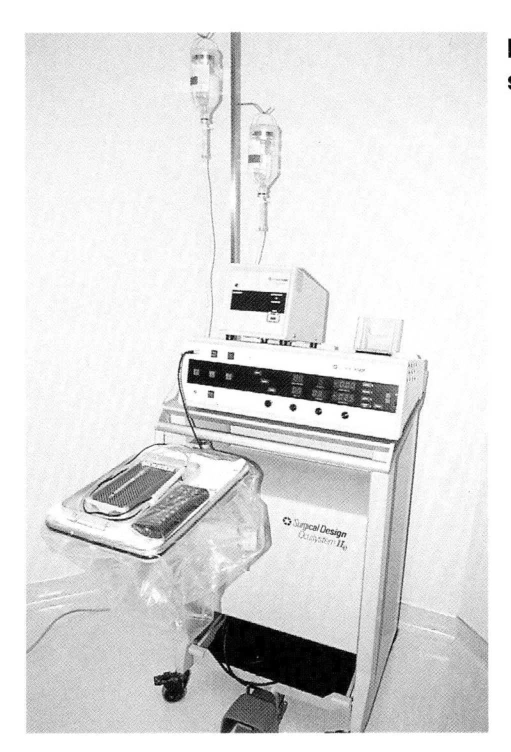

Figure 7-1. Surgical Design Ocusystem II^{art} fully set up.

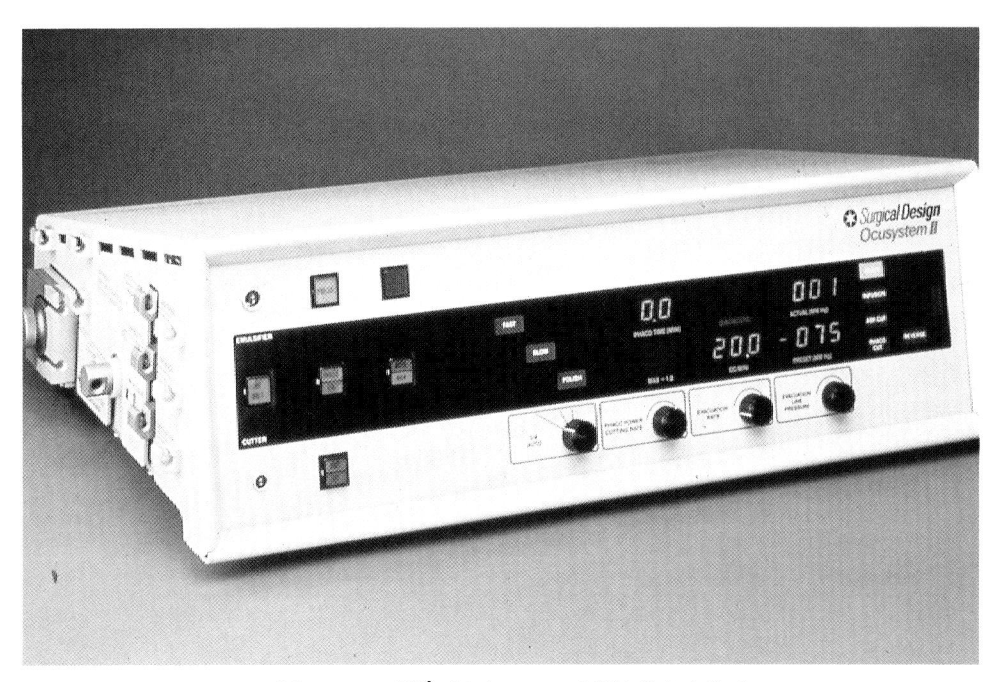

Figure 7-2. Main console of Ocusystem II^{art} with front panel LED digital display.

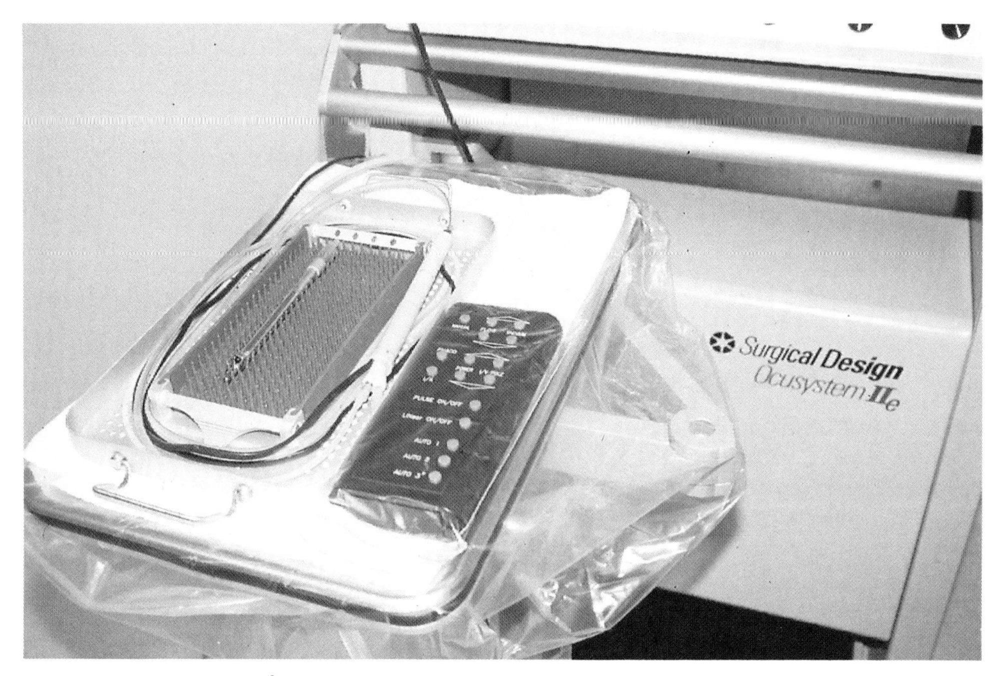

Figure 7-3. Ocusystem II^{art} instrument tray on attached articulated swing arm.

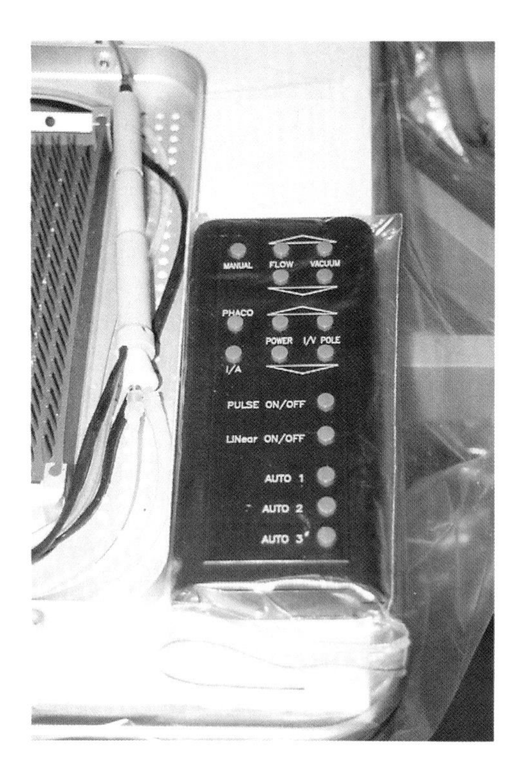

Figure 7-4. Close-up of Ocusystem II^{art} wireless remote control in sterile plastic wrap.

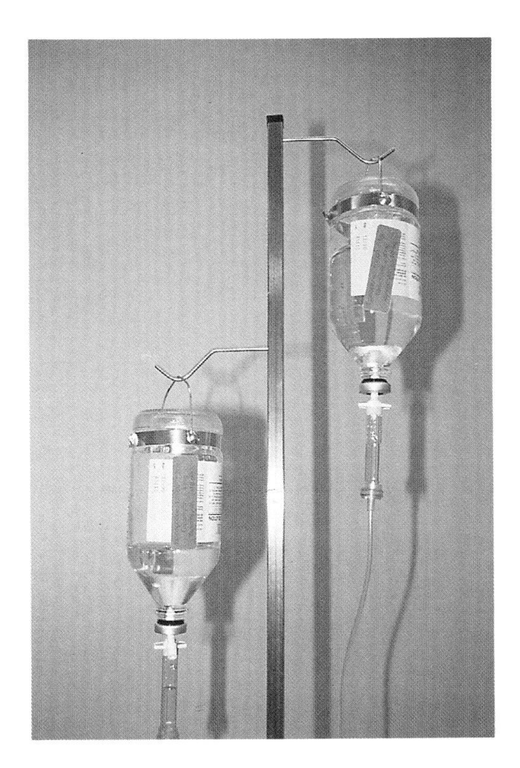

Figure 7-5. Ocusystem II^{art} double-bottle set-up for the Surge Prevention fluid venting system.

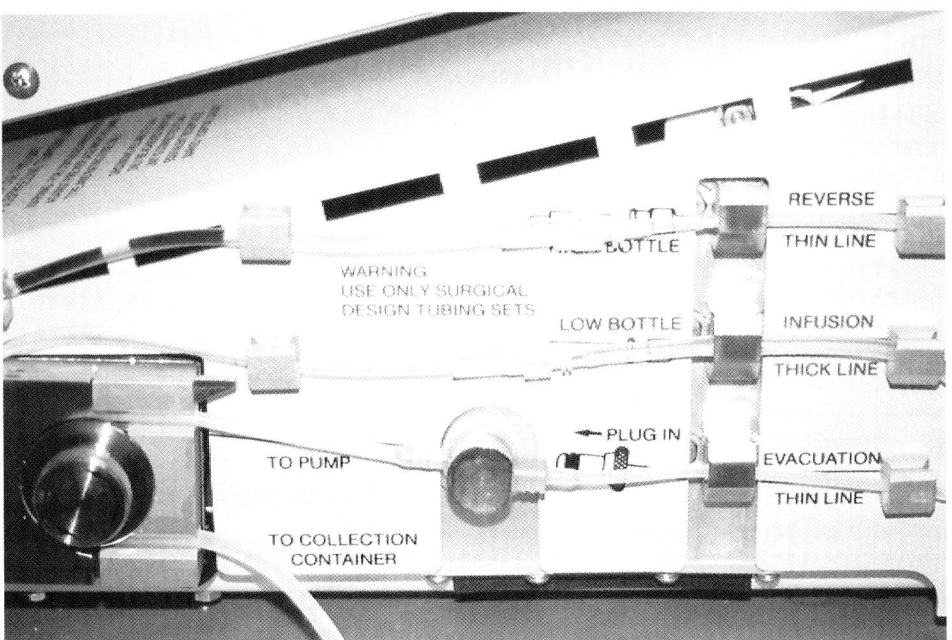

Figure 7-6. Side view of Ocusystem II^{art} main console demonstrating user-friendly silicone tubing set-up, Surge Prevention transducer and valve, and peristaltic pump pinch-roller assembly.

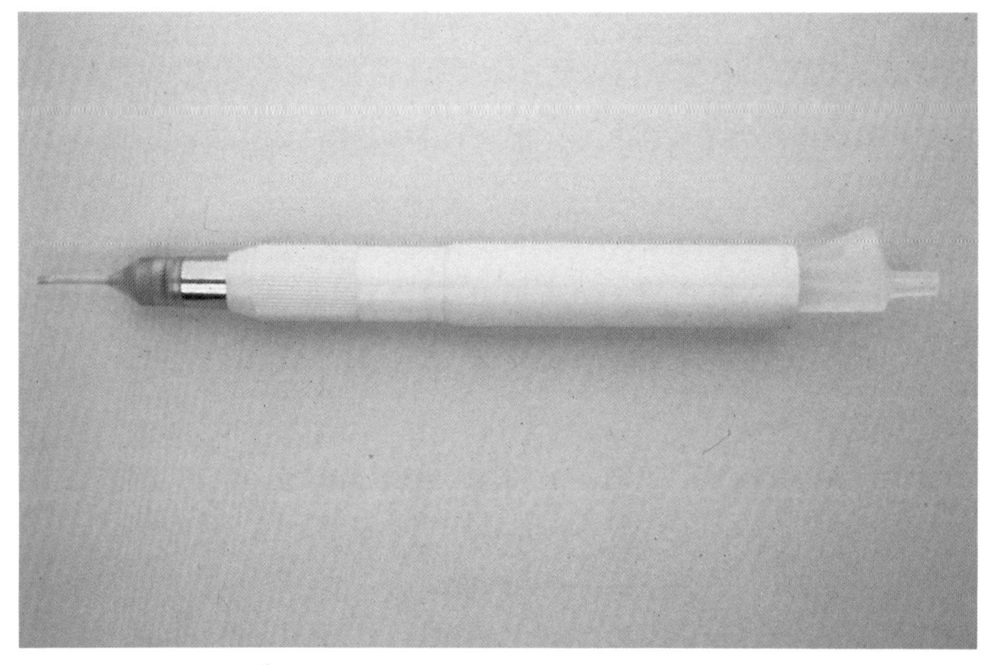

Figure 7-7. Ocusystem II^{art} "STM" lightweight plastic magnetostrictive handpiece, 5 inches in length, 1.6 oz. in weight.

upper two lines are for inflow. The top line goes to the higher of the two bottles for gravity feed for reflux and surge prevention. The middle line goes to the lower bottle for irrigation through the infusion sleeves of the phaco and I/A tips. The bottom of the three lines is for evacuation. This line first passes through the pressure transducer for the surge prevention system. It then passes over the six-pin peristaltic pump system of rollers, the speed of which is determined by the aspiration flow setting. This line passes, finally, into a collection bag.

The Handpiece

The phacoemulsification handpiece may be the smallest and lightest on the market having a plastic outer sleeve (Figure 7-7), measuring 5 inches in length and weighing only 1.6 oz. Unlike most other handpieces that are piezo-electric, this one is magnetostrictive. The original magnetostrictive handpieces contained a series of stacked metal discs. They were inefficient, ran hot, and often lost their proper resonant tuning. This generation of magnetostrictive handpieces, offered by Surgical Design, is extremely durable. The crystal in piezo-electric models vibrates in response to changes in polarity of electric current directly in contact with it. The

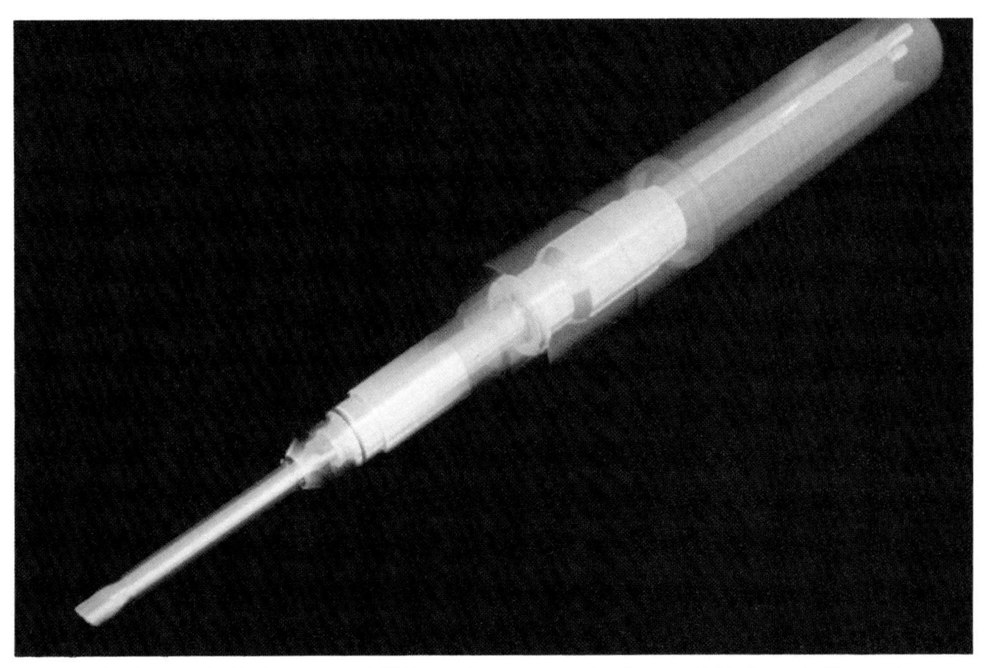

Figure 7-8. "X-ray view" diagram of STM handpiece, demonstrating straight-through-the-center aspiration for efficiency and cooling.

crystal is fragile and, therefore, most piezo-elective handpieces last for about 1000 cases. The current Surgical Design magnetostrictive handpieces have been known to last for up to 10,000 cases.[5] The previous problem of heating with earlier magnetostrictive models has been obviated by Surgical Design by running the evacuation line through the middle of the stack. This not only brings fluid to the stack for cooling, but also provides straight-line evacuation for more efficiency and less chance of occlusion (Figure 7-8).

The Cobra Tip

The traditional design of most phaco tips is to resemble a straight, hollow needle with uniform outside and inside diameters throughout the entire length of the shaft. What most manufacturers offer is a variety of different angles to the beveled tips and shafts of different diameters and shapes. Surgical Design manufactures these traditional "phaco needles" also; however, one of their most unique innovations is the design of their Cobra Tips. These tips are so named because they resemble the shape of a cobra snake with its hood expanded. The shafts of these tips are

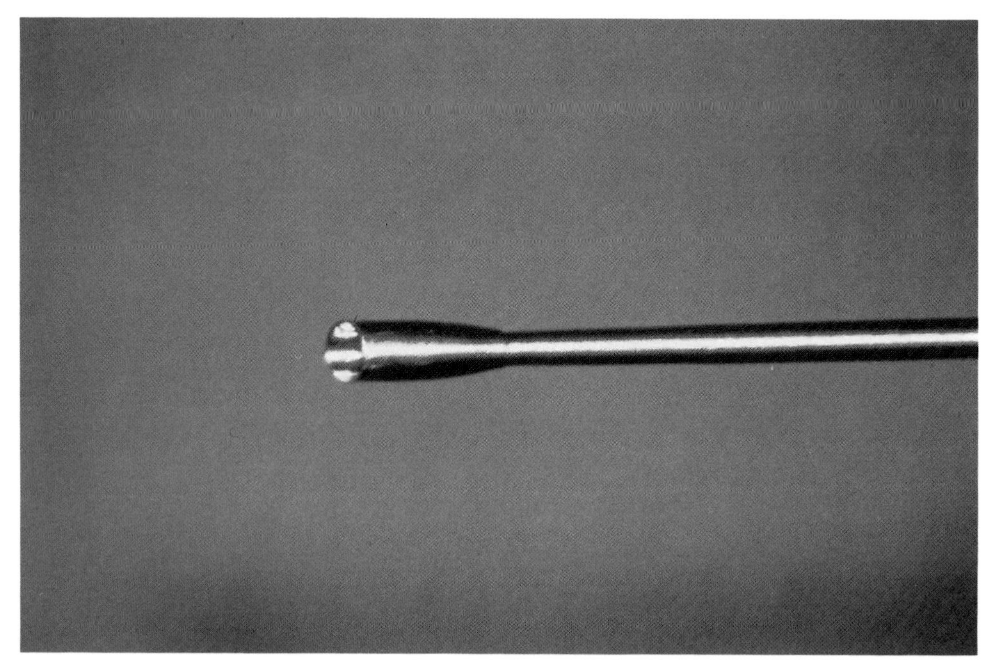

Figure 7-9. Surgical Design Cobra Tip, wide distally, narrow proximally, with funnel-shaped acoustic orifice.

not uniform throughout their entire length as are the conventional tips. Rather, they are wide distally and narrow proximally (Figure 7-9). The inner wall of the expanded distal end of the Cobra Tip is not parallel to the outer wall as in conventional tips; rather, the inner wall tapers with a shallow curve, resembling the bell end of a stethoscope (Figure 7-10). This inner bell or funnel configuration provides much more surface area for acoustic wave generation than conventional thin-walled tips and, in addition, focuses the reflected ultrasonic energy to a more concentrated area (Figures 7-11A and 7-11B). This focused delivery of ultrasound allows the surgeon to reduce the energy setting on the machine, thereby reducing nuclear "chatter," improving holding ability, enhancing the efficiency of emulsification, and reducing potential ultrasonic damage to the surrounding tissues, such as the corneal endothelium.

The Cobra Tip is presently manufactured in two readily available sizes, although Surgical Design can make tips almost any size to suit the surgeon's preference. The "Maxi" version is designed to be used through a 2.65-mm incision, while the "Mini" is for 2.5-mm incisions. The larger Maxi Tip is smaller than most standard tips in use today, which require a 3.0- or 3.2-mm incision. This is a particular advan-

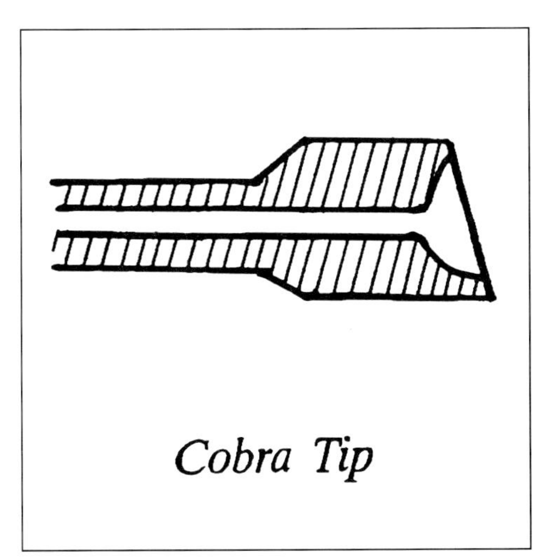

Figure 7-10. Cross-sectional diagram of Surgical Design Cobra Tip demonstrating wide distal shaft, narrow proximal shaft, and funnel-shaped orifice.

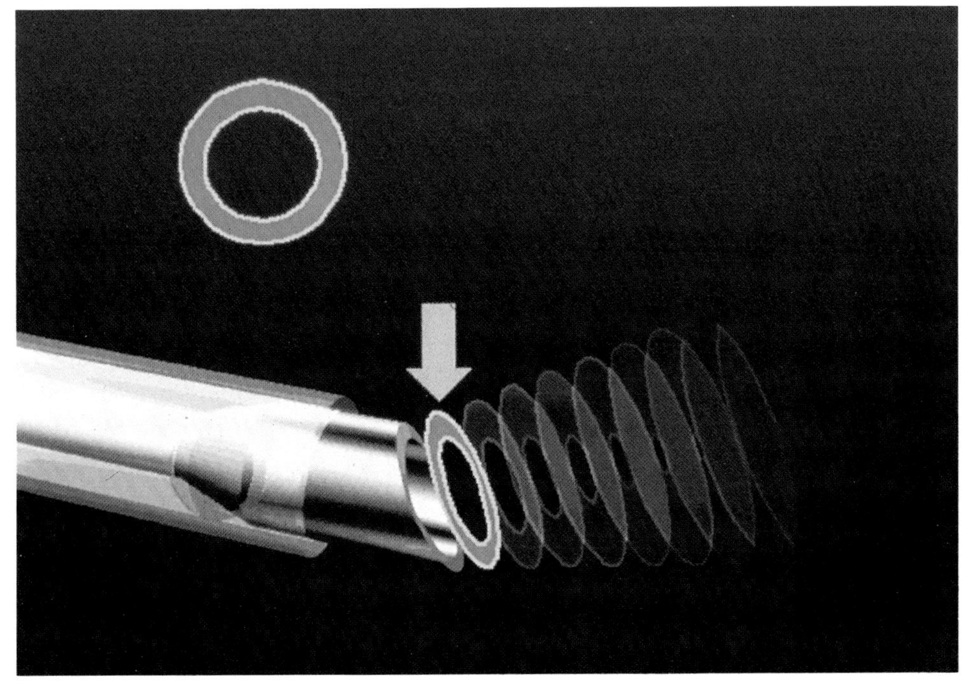

Figure 7-11A. Acoustic wave form generated by peripheral ring of ordinary phaco tips.

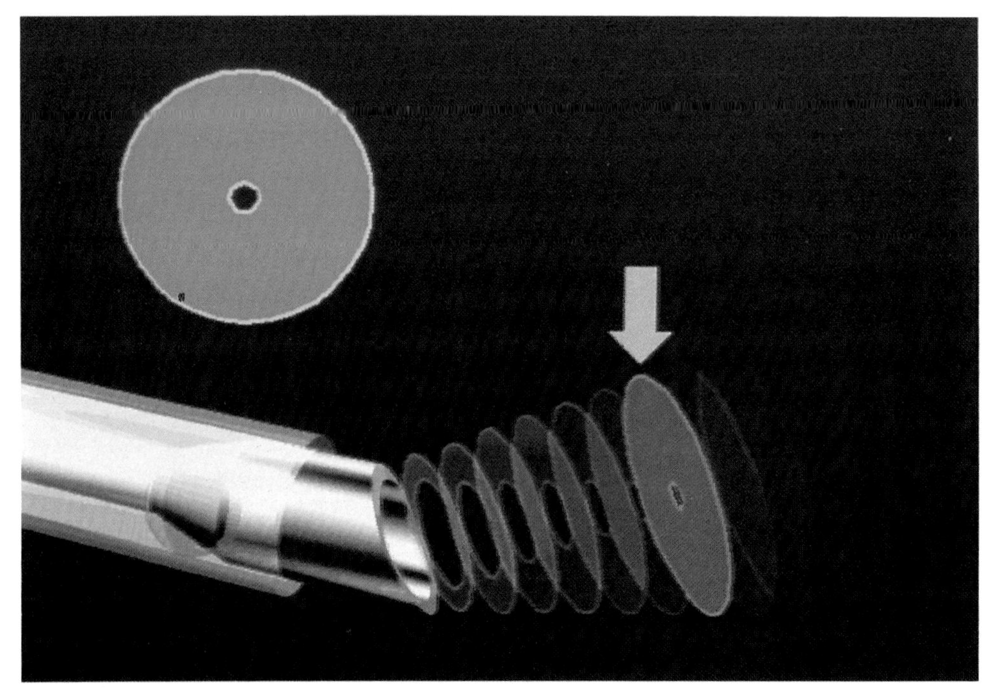

Figure 7-11B. Acoustic wave form generated by Cobra Tip funnel design.

tage in sutureless clear-corneal surgery where "smaller is better."[6] The Maxi Cobra has a shaft internal diameter (ID) of approximately 0.8 mm, while the Mini's ID is approximately 0.6 mm. While these smaller diameter phaco tips have the advantage of usability through smaller incisions, they also carry the disadvantages of requiring slightly more time, as they cut smaller paths and remove less volume of nucleus with each pass, and they have a slightly greater tendency to clog, which can be minimized by higher aspiration and vacuum levels.

Surgical Design phaco tips are available with standard plastic sleeves or metal sleeves. The plastic phaco sleeves are of rigid, clear polysulfone (Figure 7-12) which are non-compressible, thereby preventing thermal tissue damage. The rigid polysulfone phaco sleeve attaches to the handpiece at the tapered base of the Cobra Tip. The space between the sleeve and the tapered base is referred to as a "protective cocoon," designed to prevent the formation of unwanted cavitation bubbles.[7]

Like the phaco tips, the I/A tips are available with either soft silicone sleeves that conform to the shape of the incision, thereby providing a seal, or with rigid

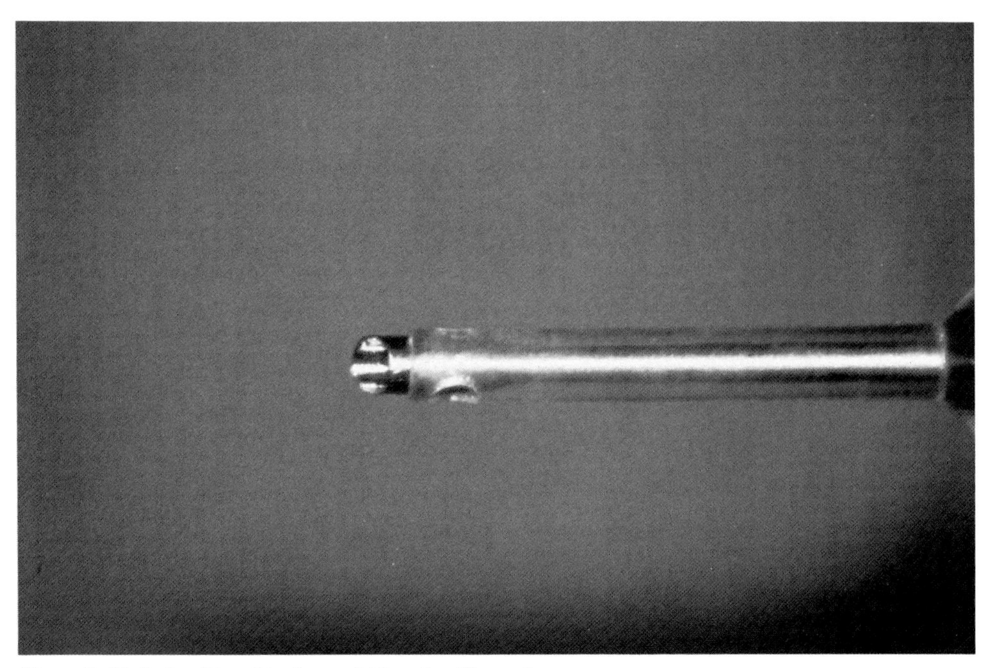

Figure 7-12. Cobra Tip with clear, rigid, polysulfone sleeve.

metal sleeves. The I/A tips are manufactured with several port sizes, 0.2, 0.3, and 0.5 mm being the most common. The I/A tips are also available in various configurations: straight, angled, J-shaped, Binkhorst, etc, and are also available for **ultrasonic I/A** for capsule polishing.

The Foot Pedal

Surgeon activation of machine functions is provided by a standard three-position foot switch (Figure 7-13 and Table 7-1). Reflux is activated by lifting the foot off the main depression pedal to position 0 and continuing to lift the foot until an upper switch is compressed. Unlike the three-position depression foot pedal, the reflux activator does not have linear control, only "on" or "off," opening a valve to the higher of the two bottles, allowing the fluid in the evacuation line to reverse direction and exit the handpiece by gravity feed.

Figure 7-13. Ocusystem II^{art} three-position foot pedal with upper reflux "kicker."

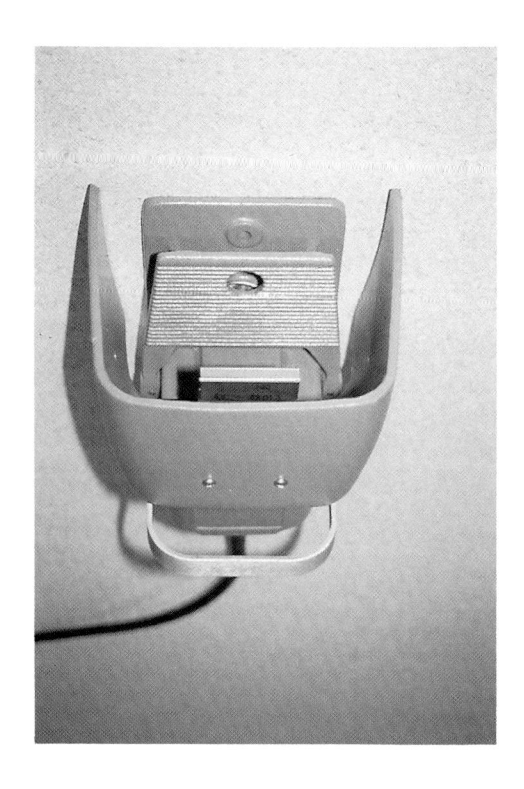

Machine Functions

Unlike machines of earlier generations, "setting the dials" on these new "high-tech" machines with chips, sensors, transducers, etc, is no longer a matter of simply selecting power, flow, and vacuum settings. As a matter of fact, with earlier machines, the surgeon could operate using "standard factory settings."

Power

With the Ocusystem II^{art}, the only function that has remained simple and unchanged is the power. The frequency is factory set at 44 kHz (44,000 cps). This does not change: this frequency begins as soon as the surgeon engages foot position 3 and remains constant throughout the entire range of this foot position. What does change, as with all machines when the phaco setting is on "linear," is the stroke length or the axial excursion of the Cobra Tip. This, as before, is under linear foot pedal control when position 3 is engaged, increasing with further depression of the pedal, reaching the preset maximum at full pedal depression. The maximum power level is set by either a dial on the front of the console or by remote control and is displayed by LED as a decimal fraction. My present power setting, for all degrees of nuclear hardness, is 0.4, 40% of the maximum stroke length of this handpiece. If the machine is set in the non-linear mode, this maximum level is present continuously anywhere in foot position 3.

It is not possible to quantitatively compare the phaco power settings of different machines, as the stroke lengths vary and, specifically with the Surgical Design machine, the Cobra Tip's delivery of ultrasonic energy is different from all other tips. As with other machines, the ultrasonic energy can be delivered in either **continuous mode** or a **pulsed mode**. Pulsed ultrasound, a feature first incorporated as a phaco function by Surgical Design, is intended to improve both attractability and holdability, especially of hard nuclear fragments. An optimal pulse rate with the Cobra Tip is around six per second.

Other convenient features of the Ocusystem II^{art} are **automatic tuning**, which occurs at the push of a button when the machine is set up, and **continuous tuning**, which maintains a constant frequency (44 kHz) moment by moment during operation, especially as the tip milieu is constantly changing, eg, from BSS to viscoelastic to nucleus.

Fluidics

Being among the current generation of machines manufactured by a company whose interest has always been serving the surgeons with ever-changing technology, and having had the elite braintrust resource in Anton Banko, Jerre Freeman, Steve Shearing, Buol Heslin, Richard Mackool, Terry Devine, Jack Singer, and others, it is not surprising that the latest model Ocusystem II^{art} would have two special fluidics features that make the machine one of the most sophisticated, safe, and efficient on the market: these are referred to as **Adjustable Rise Time** and **Surge Prevention.**

Adjustable Rise Time

This is the newest feature to be designed into the Ocusystem II^{art}. Its purpose is to further refine surgeon control, flexibility, efficiency, and safety during the stages of nuclear removal. Vacuum, as a function, has two controllable variables: the upper limit and the rate of rise. As with other machines, the surgeon first selects the upper limit of vacuum, which ranges from 15 to 500 mmHg. With peristaltic pumps, the aspiration flow rate, as determined by the pump speed, determines the rate of rise of the vacuum when the tip is occluded. At low flow, it may take 3 to 4 seconds for the vacuum to reach 150 mmHg, while at higher flow, it may take only 1 second.

With previous generations of peristaltic machines, the flow rate (pump speed) and, consequently, the rate of rise of the vacuum remained constant throughout the entire period of occlusion. With the new Adjustable Rise Time feature of the Ocusystem II[art], the surgeon can select a point along the vacuum curve at which the rate of rise will automatically change. This rate-of-rise change occurs as a result of an automatic preset change in the flow rate or pump speed, thereby creating a bimodal, biphasic, or two-stage rate of rise in the vacuum. This has particular value when removing pieces of nucleus at high flow and vacuum. For example, the flow may be set at 24 cc/min and the vacuum at 110 mmHg. The initial flow rate of 24 cc/min pulls the quadrants to the Cobra Tip and the vacuum begins to rise rapidly upon occlusion, establishing a firm hold on the piece of nucleus for emulsification. The Adjustable Rise Time can slow the flow, say, to 8 cc/min when the vacuum reaches a point midway up, say, 60 mmHg (Figure 7-14). By slowing the flow rate at 60 mmHg of vacuum, the maximum vacuum limit of 110 mmHg is then approached

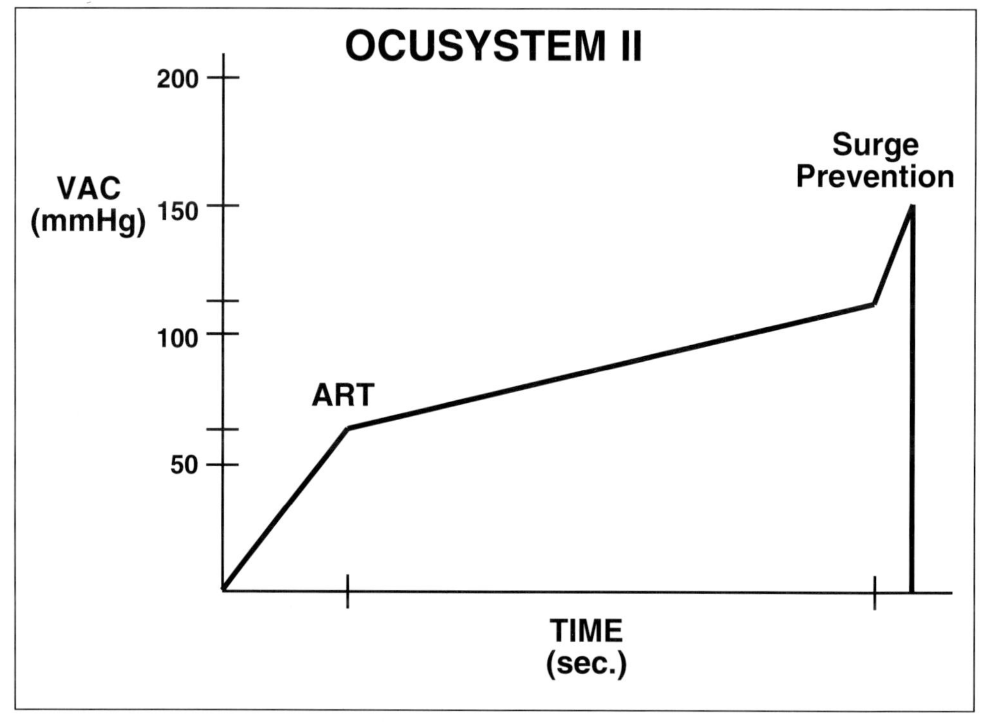

Figure 7-14. Two-stage vacuum rate of rise with the Adjustable Rise Time (ART) set to slow the flow at 60 mmHg vacuum. Surge Prevention mechanism set to drop vacuum to zero at approximately 140 mmHg.

more slowly and, hence, more safely.

The surgeon may alternatively prefer to increase the flow rate to, perhaps, 30 cc/min instead, in order to speed up the process of emulsification and evacuation at the Cobra Tip.

Surge Prevention

The Surge Prevention feature is designed to save capsules and irises. The concept is based upon the phenomenon known to all phaco surgeons as vacuum surge. When a piece of nuclear material is held on the phaco tip for a few moments, the vacuum begins to rise in the tubing, handpiece, and phaco tip. When the piece is sufficiently emulsified and the vacuum has risen high enough to overcome the resistance, a critical point is reached at which the material is suddenly aspirated into the tip. With the phaco tip no longer occluded, the high vacuum is immediately transferred toward the intraocular environment. Within a fraction of a second, faster than humans can react, the intraocular contents are drawn toward the phaco tip by the high vacuum, risking damage to the capsule, vitreous, iris, and cornea.

The pressure transducer that is incorporated into the Ocusystem II^{art} senses such sudden elevations in vacuum pressure and automatically opens a valve, immediately connecting the fluid in the high bottle to the evacuation line. This gravity-fed infusion fluid is rapidly drawn into the evacuation tubing by the high vacuum, instantly neutralizing the vacuum, resulting in immediate stabilization of the anterior chamber (see Figure 7-14).

The vacuum level at which this valve opens is programmable with a dial on the back of the console. Surgeons are now using techniques, such as Phaco Chop,[8] that require greater attractability and holdability. They are, therefore, raising both the flow and vacuum levels to as much as 30 cc/min and 500 mmHg.[9,10] Both the Surge Prevention features of this machine and the Adjustable Rise Time provide added safety for these high-flow, high-vacuum techniques.

Machine Settings

Like all of the current machines described in this text, the Ocusystem II^{art} has both **automatic** and **manual** settings. In the manual mode, any parameter may be entered at any time during the procedure, giving the surgeon virtually infinite flexibility and control, and without disturbing the previously programmed automatic settings. Three sets of automatic parameters are programmable for both phaco (Table 7-2) and I/A. In this way, one surgeon may use all three for different stages of the procedure or for different degrees of nuclear hardness, or the three different settings may be used for three different surgeons. The Ocusystem II[art] has the added convenience of instant changeability from one auto setting to another without requiring the surgeon to lift his or her foot off the foot pedal, and this can be accomplished on command by the surgical assistant with a touch of the finger on the remote control.

Phacoemulsification Technique

After making a 2.65-mm clear-corneal incision with a trapezoid diamond blade (Figure 7-15), the Maxi Cobra Tip is inserted into the incision bevel-down with reflux on (Figure 7-16). The tip is then rotated in the incision to bevel-up position (Figure 7-17) and is advanced into the anterior chamber (Figure 7-18). Sculpting of the primary groove is begun (Figure 7-19) on phaco setting Auto 1, flow 8 cc/min, vacuum

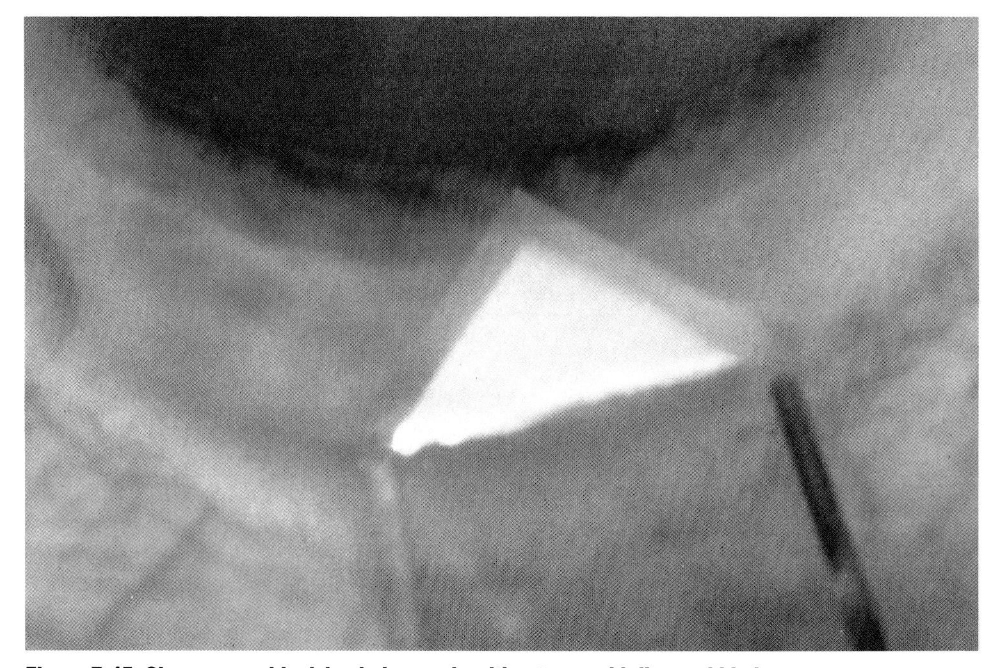

Figure 7-15. Clear-corneal incision being made with a trapezoid diamond blade.

25 mmHg, and power 0.4 (40%). This very low-flow, low-vacuum setting produces an extremely stable anterior chamber and allows for phaco to occur safely in the presence of small pupils and shallow chambers.

Following primary grooving, additional grooves may be created (Figure 7-20) for four-quadrant technique or no further grooving if Phaco Chop is to be performed. After grooving, I request the sterile technician change the phaco settings to Auto 3, raising the flow to 24 cc/min and the vacuum to 110 mmHg, leaving the power still at 0.4 (40%). The Adjustable Rise Time is set to automatically change the flow from 24 cc/min to 8 cc/min when the vacuum level reaches 60 mmHg. The Surge Prevention valve is set to open and drop the vacuum to zero at approximately 140 mmHg. Fracturing is then performed with two instruments (Figure 7-21) and the quadrant to be removed is elevated with the secondhand instrument, a blunt Barraquer iris spatula (Figure 7-22). The quadrants are then aspirated to the Cobra Tip, held in occlusion, and safely emulsified (Figure 7-23) with the extra protection of the Adjustable Rise Time and Surge Prevention functions.

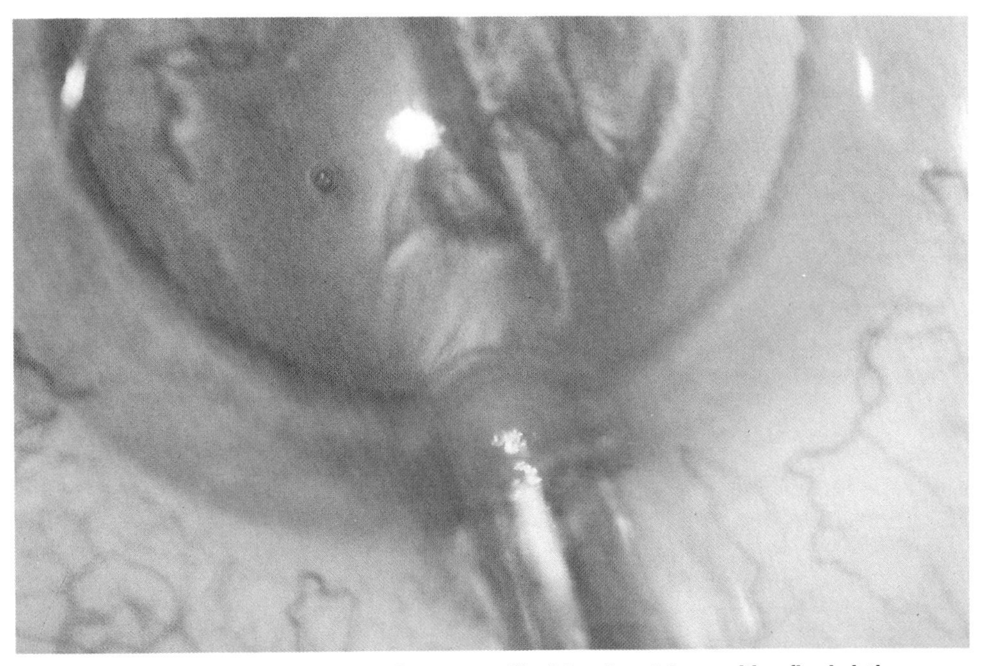

Figure 7-16. Cobra Tip introduced into clear-corneal incision, bevel down, with reflux irriation.

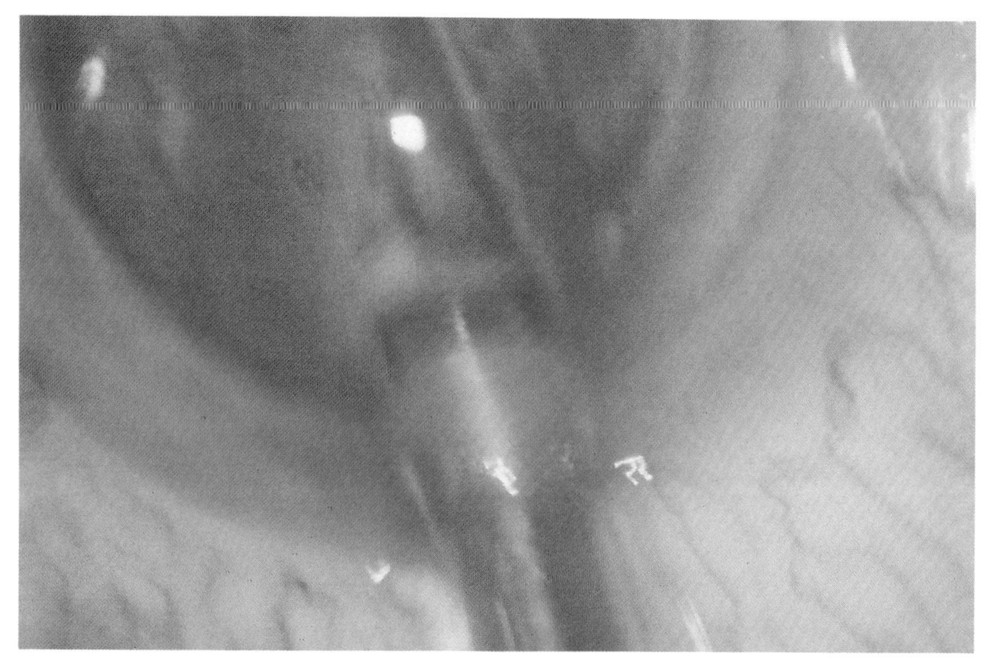

Figure 7-17. Cobra Tip in clear-corneal incision with bevel rotated up.

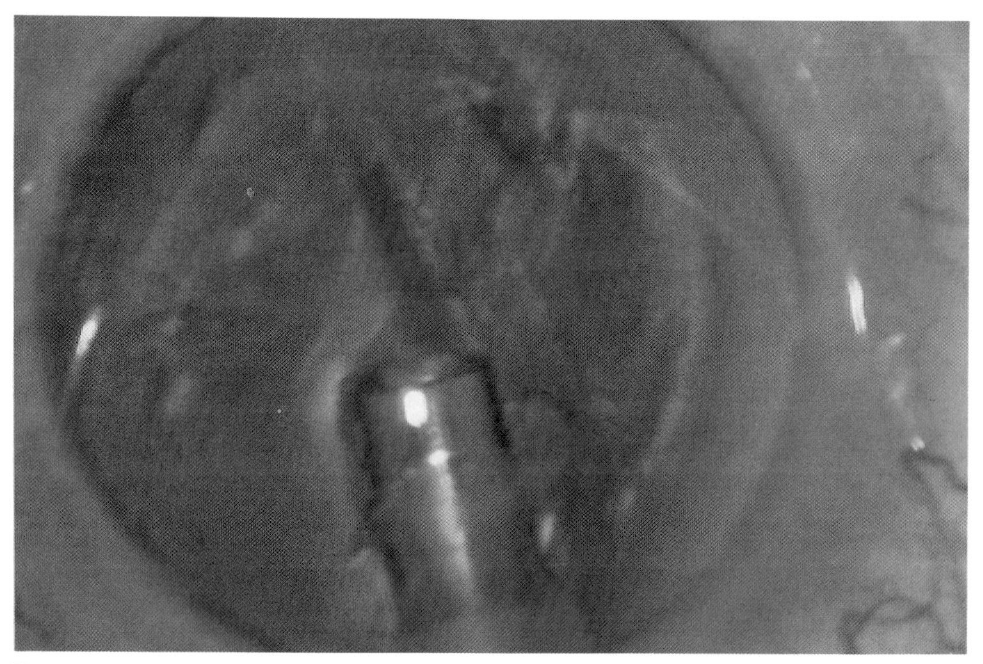

Figure 7-18. Cobra Tip advanced into anterior chamber now with sleeve irrigation (foot position 1).

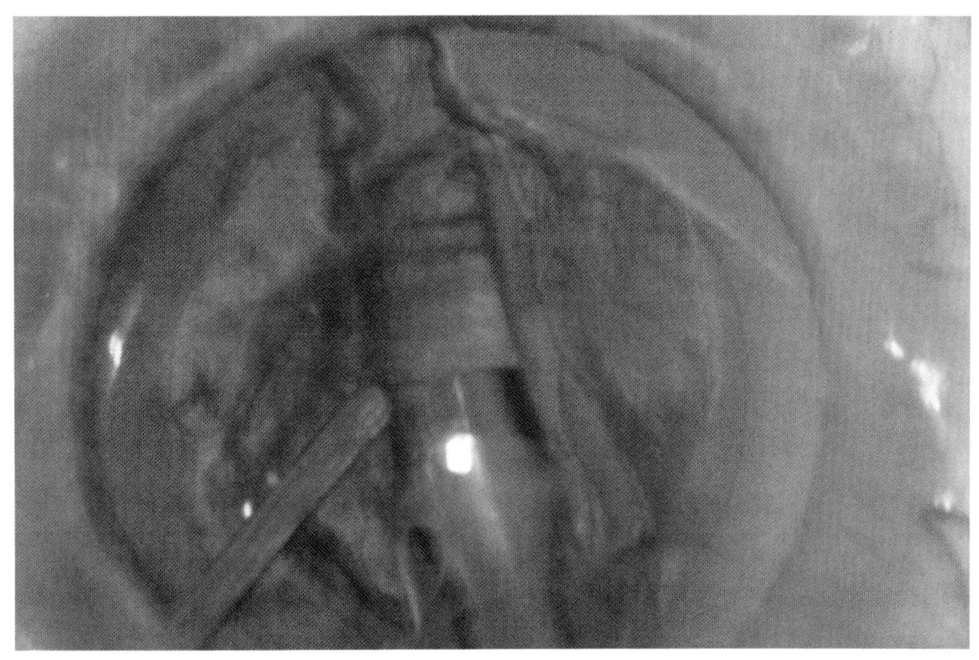

Figure 7-19. Primary groove sculpting on Auto 1 setting: low flow of 8 cc/min, low vacuum of 25 mmHg, and low power of 0.4 (40%).

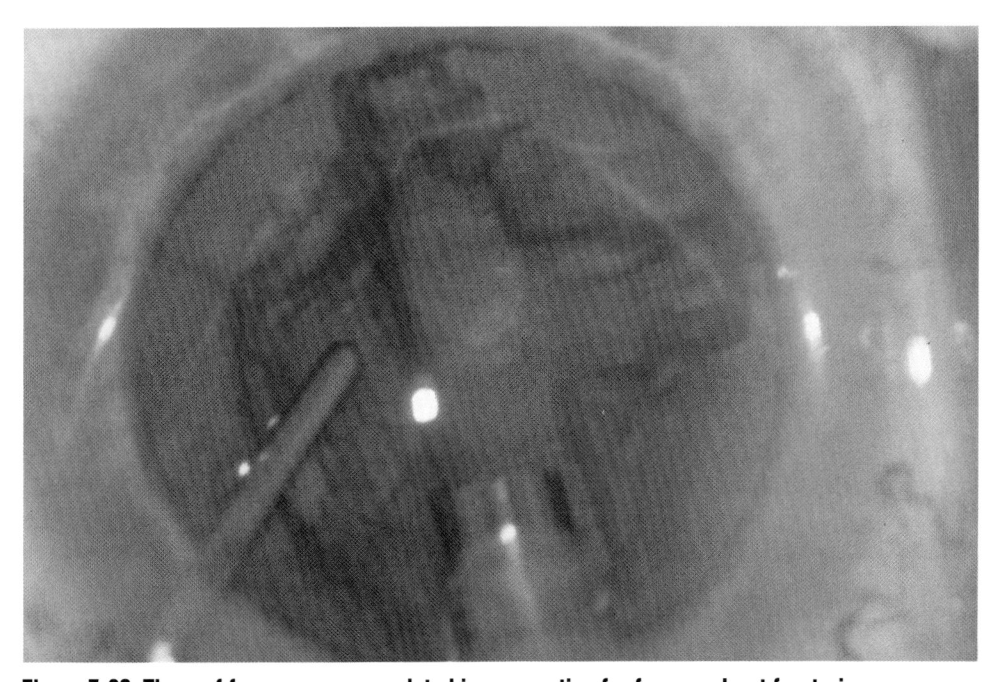

Figure 7-20. Three of four grooves completed in preparation for four-quadrant fracturing.

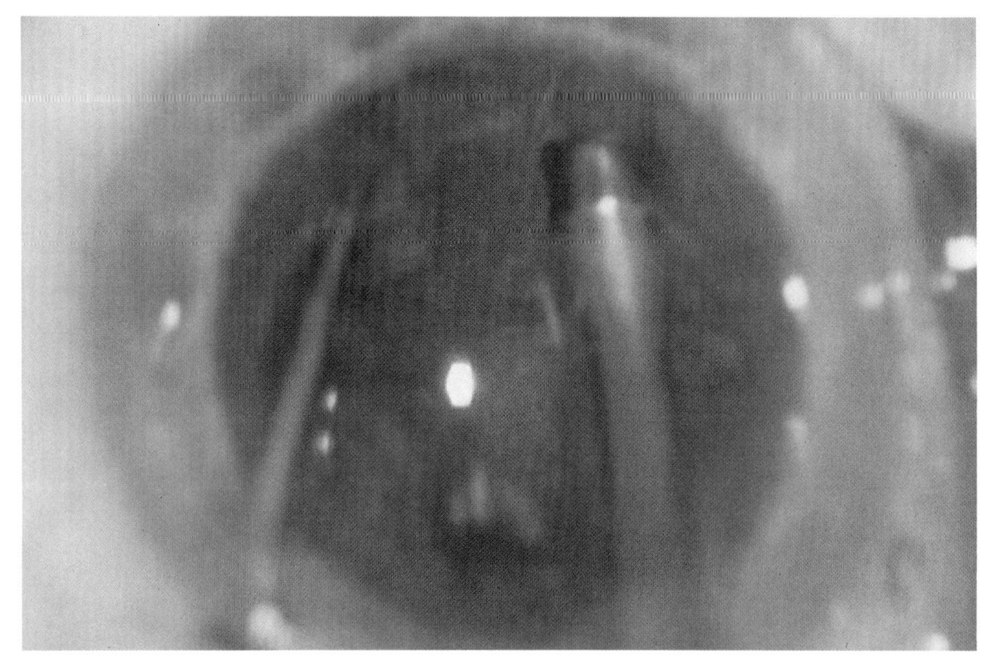

Figure 7-21. Bimanual fracturing using the Cobra Tip and a Barraquer iris spatula (Storz, #E485).

Irrigation/Aspiration

I/A flow and vacuum levels are also programmable into the three Auto settings. I remove remaining cortex **after** cortical-cleaving viscodissection and IOL implantation (Figure 7-24), using low-flow and high-vacuum. The foot pedal actually is programmed to operate in three stages during I/A (Table 7-3), just as during phaco. In foot position 2, the flow is 8 cc/min and the vacuum begins at 150 mmHg for slow and safe engagement of cortex. Once the I/A tip is occluded and the cortex begins to strip away from the capsule, the I/A tip is moved centrally, safely over the IOL optic. The foot pedal is then depressed maximally in position 3, raising the vacuum to 450 mmHg, giving more "pulling power" to the tip to clear the cortical fragment.

Auto 2 is set for slightly higher flow, 12 cc/min, to improve attractability, and **Auto 3** is for vacuuming the capsule with very low flow, 2 cc/min, and very low vacuum, 15 mmHg.

I have recently added tips with 0.2-mm ports which are slower at removing the cortex than 0.3-mm tips, but are more effective at removing small strands of cortical fibers, sometimes referred to as "seaweed."

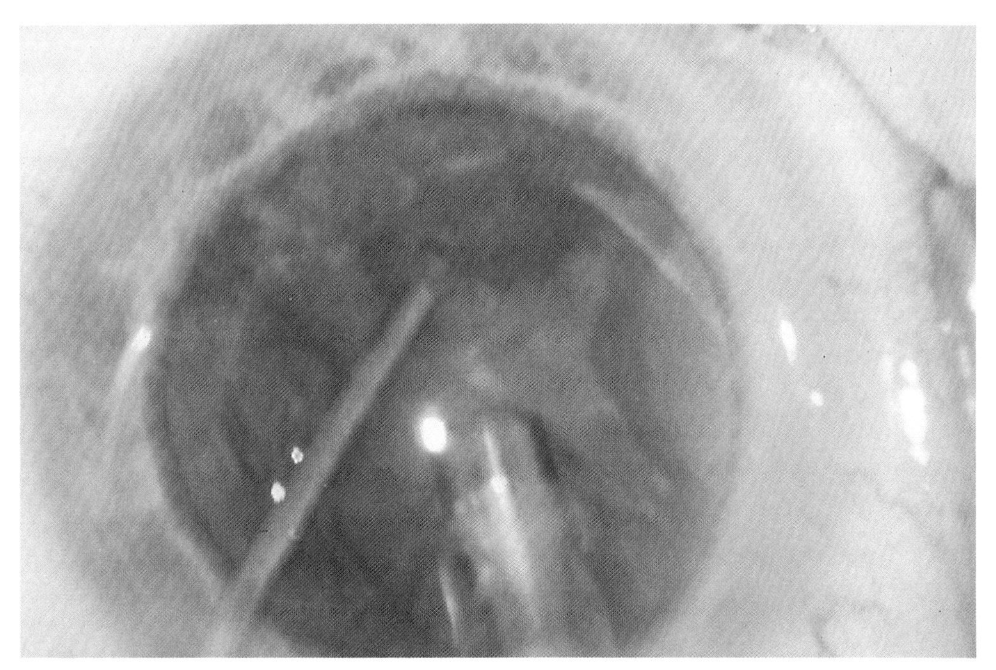

Figure 7-22. Elevation of first quadrant at its apex in preparation for emulsification.

Vitrectomy

The Ocusystem II^{art} vitrectomy unit has physically been separated from the phacoemulsification console. It is called the Ocutine and, in our operating rooms, rests on top of the Ocusystem II^{art} console (Figure 7-25). Both guillotine and rotary cutters are available, although most surgeons now prefer the former. The cutting rate is set by a dial from 180 cuts/min to 600 cuts/min (Table 7-4).

For automated anterior vitrectomy, the bottle is lowered until the flow from the vitrectomy tip is at a rapid drip. The flow is slow at 6 cc/min, the vacuum limit is set at 150 mmHg, and the cut rate at 300 cuts/min, which is "0.5" as displayed on the console. The irrigation sleeve is not removed for separation of infusion and aspiration; rather, the infusion line is pinched in the left hand while "dry" vitrectomy is performed with the right hand. The infusion line is unpinched (opened) only for incremental fluid maintenance of the anterior chamber. In this way, continuous sideport infusion with possible hydration of the vitreous is avoided.

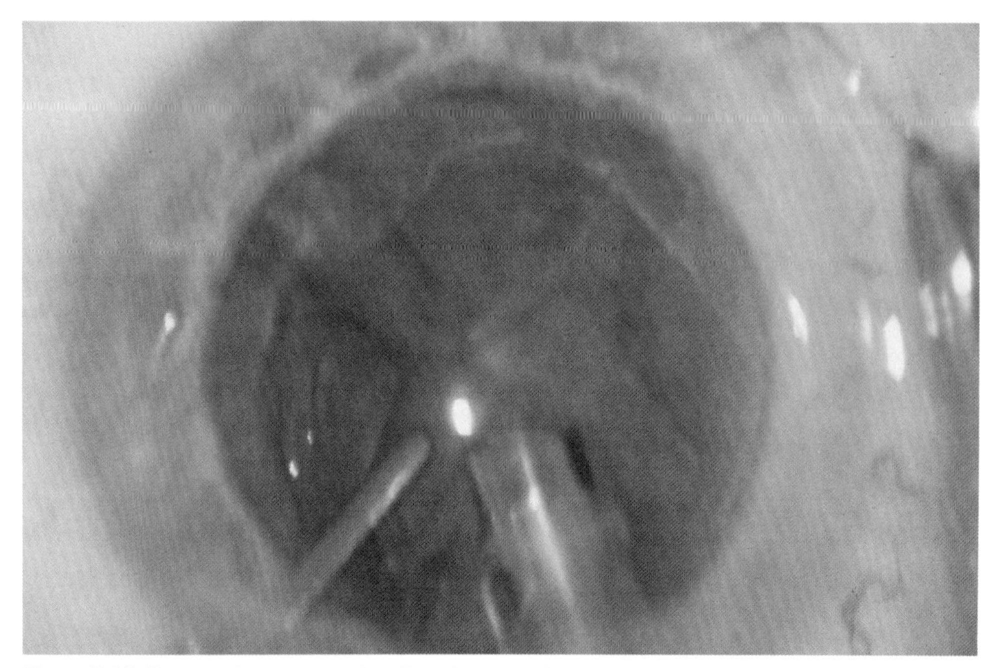

Figure 7-23. First quadrant removed on Auto 3 setting: flow 24 cc/min, vacuum 110 mmHg, power 0.4 (40%), ART 8 cc @ 60 mmHg, and Surge Prevention 140 mmHg.

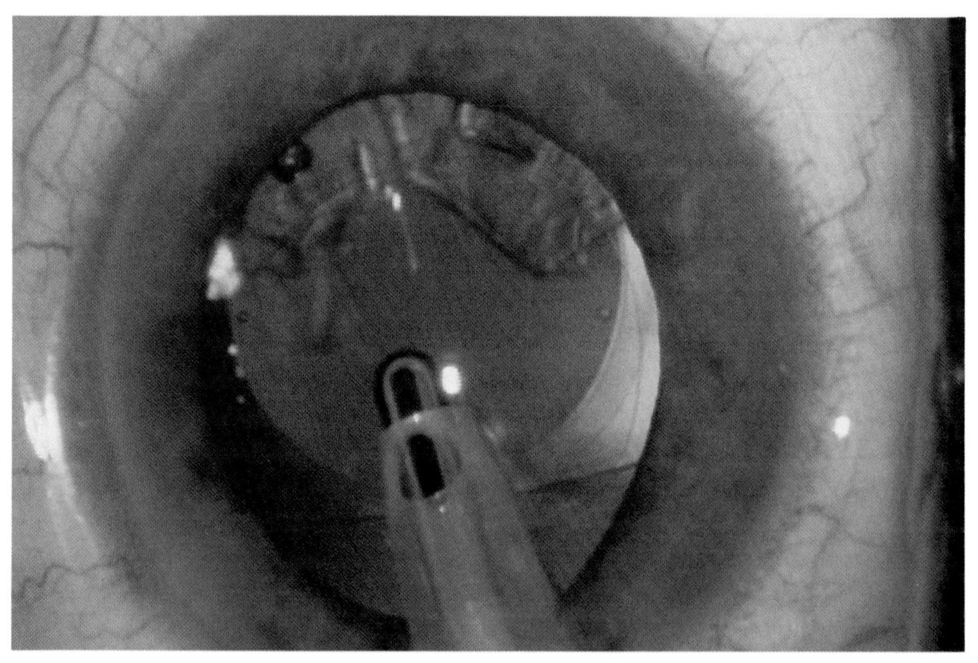

Figure 7-24. Post-implantation cortical aspiration on Auto 1: flow 8 cc/min and two-stage vacuum 150/450 mmHg.

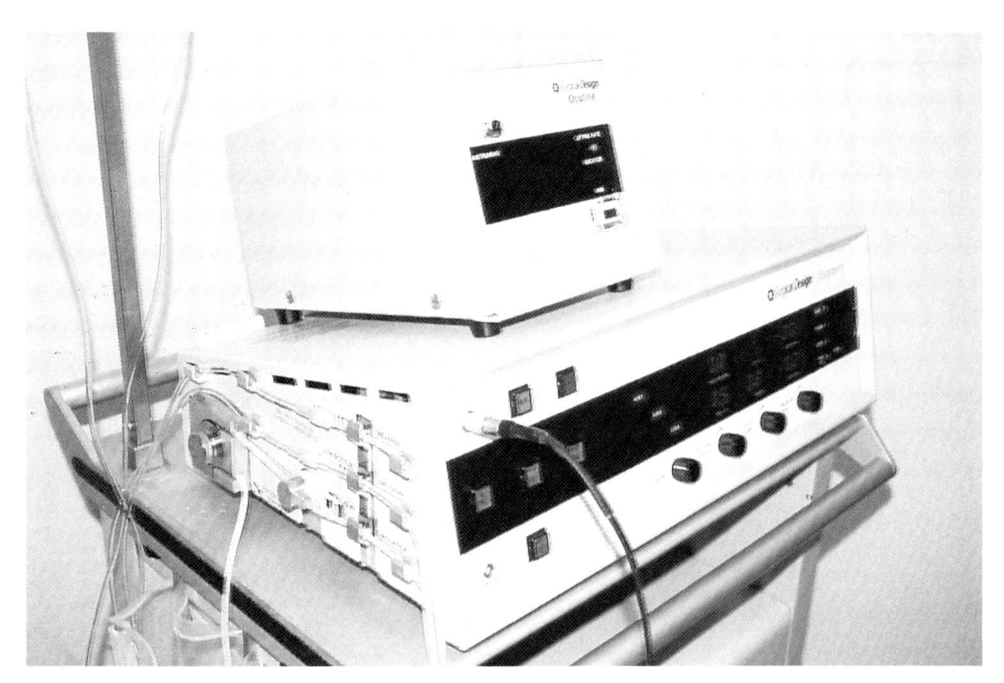

Figure 7-25. Surgical Design Ocutine automated vitrectomy unit atop the Ocusystem II^{art} console.

A Personal Choice

In October 1994, I opened the Center for Advanced Eye Surgery, a new two-operating room ambulatory surgical facility attached to the Sarasota Cataract Institute. After performing phacoemulsification and foldable lens implantation for 7 years, I was interested in a phaco machine that would have ultimate programmability, would have the latest features for safety, would be ergonomically user-friendly, and would perform phaco through smaller and smaller incisions. As many of the readers know, my cataract technique has evolved to clear-corneal incision. In the cornea, it appears that incisions of 2.5 mm approach true astigmatic neutrality and possess a tensile strength that would satisfy Paul Ernest. The Ocusystem II^{art} Mini Cobra Tip fits safely through a 2.5 mm incision, and Jim Carty has demonstrated that the plate-haptic silicone IOL can be inserted through incisions as small as 1.5 mm.[11] This got my attention.

The unique design of the Cobra Tip, efficiently emulsifying at greatly reduced power, and the clear, rigid sleeve eliminating corneal burn potential, were attractive features. The lightweight plastic phaco handpiece reduced hand fatigue and added a new level of gentleness and delicateness to finger movements. The advanced fluidics, with Adjustable Rise Time and Surge Prevention features, enhanced my confidence in the machine. Finally, the reusable tubing made it an economically prudent investment in light of the current managed care environment.

Acknowledgments

I would like to acknowledge Sharon Martell at the Sarasota Cataract Institute for her efficient preparation of this manuscript. I would also like to express my appreciation to Terry Devine, MD, Jack Singer, MD, and William Banko, MD, for their educational and technical contributions, without which this chapter could not have been written.

Table 7-1. Surgical Design Ocusystem II^{art} Foot Pedal Functions

Foot Position	Phaco	I/A	Vitrectomy
1	Irrigation	Irrigation	Irrigation
2	Irrigation Aspiration	Irrigation Aspiration Vacuum Level 1	Irrigation Aspiration
3	Irrigation Aspiration Emulsification	Irrigation Aspiration Vacuum Level 2	Irrigation Aspiration Cutting

Table 7-2. Dr. Grabow's Example of Three Phacoemulsification Auto Settings for Surgical Design Ocusystem II^art

Function	Setting	Phaco
Sculpting	Auto 1 (ART)	8/25 (4 @ 30)
Quadrant Removal	Auto 2 (ART)	24/140 (8 @ 80)
Quadrant Removal	Auto 3 (ART)	24/110 (8 @ 60)

Table 7-3. Dr. Grabow's Irrigation/Aspiration Settings for Surgical Design Ocusystem II^art

I/A Setting	Flow	Vacuum
Auto 1	8	150 (Foot Position 2) 450 (Foot Position 3)
Auto 2	12	150 (Foot Position 2) 450 (Foot Position 3)
Auto 3	2	15

Table 7-4. Surgical Design Ocusystem II^art Ocutine Automated Vitrectomy Cutting Rate Settings

Settings	Cuts/Minute
0.3	180
0.4	240
0.5	300
0.6	360
0.7	420
0.8	480
0.9	540
1.0	600

References

1. Surgical Design monograph. *A Company History—DRG Series.* Surgical Design Corporate History (Surgical Design Corp, 4253—21st St, LIC, NY 11101): Volume 2, Series 2.
2. Banko A. Dynamics of intraocular flow and ultrasound power. *Ocular Surgery News.* May 1, 1986.
3. Freeman JM. Silicone tubing effective but requires meticulous cleaning. *Ocular Surgery News.* Dec 15, 1986.
4. Surgical Design monograph. *Tubing Measurements and Selections.* (Surgical Design Corp, 4253—21st St, LIC, NY 11101): Sept 17, 1993.
5. Devine TM. Phaco: evolution without hard data. *Ocular Surgery News.* Sept 1, 1993;II.
6. Ernest PH, Lavery KT, Kiessling LA. Relative strength of scleral corneal and clear corneal incision constructed in cadaver eyes. *J Cataract Refract Surg.* 1994;20:626-629.
7. Singer JA. Funnel-shaped tip controls ultrasound energy during phaco. *Ocular Surgery News.* Jul 1, 1992.
8. Nagahara KB. Advanced phaco-chop technique boosts safety, cuts ultrasound time for hard nuclei. *Ocular Surgery News.* Feb 1, 1995.
9. Singer JA. High-vacuum phaco system allows better intraocular control. *Ophthalmology Times.* Sept 15, 1994;19.
10. Devine TM. Preferred technique employs high-vacuum. *Ocular Surgery News.* Sept 15, 1994;12.
11. Carty JB. The littlest cataract/IOL—surgeon stretches limit of lens insertion. *Ocular Surgery News.* Mar 1, 1994.

Chapter 8

PhacoTmesis

Aziz Anis, MD

PhacoTmesis, manufactured by Chiron Vision, is not and has never been meant to be just another phacoemulsification machine (Figures 8-1 through 8-3). Currently, there are enough phaco machines on the market that are extremely efficient, with highly sophisticated fluidics systems that cater to every whim and desire of the modern cataract surgeon. Not only has the technology in design and manufacture of phacoemulsification machines advanced so impressively during the past 25 years, ever since Kelman introduced his revolutionary concept, but also pioneers of the operation from Kratz and Sinskey to Gimbel, Fine, and Nagahara have revolutionized the technique. These remarkable surgeons, with a host of equally talented others, have continued to refine and fine-tune the techniques of phacoemulsification to an extremely high level of precision, predictability, and safety.

However, the safety features of any of these machines utilizing any of these advanced techniques of phacoemulsification depends primarily and totally on the surgeon in choosing the proper parameters of the machine for each patient and each technique. Performing the procedure with undivided attention and concentration and a substantial level of skill to permit him or her to remove all the contents of the capsular bag without ever touching the posterior or anterior capsular membrane or the iris with the activated ultrasonic tip is also critical. If the activated tip touches

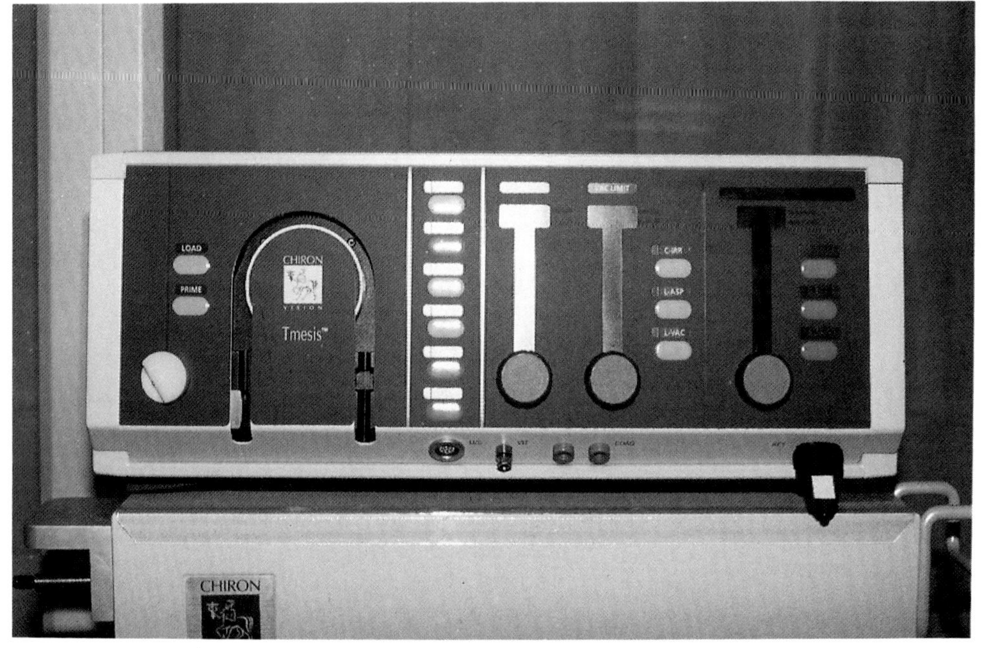

Figure 8-1. Chiron PhacoTmesis Machine.

any of these structures, damage will happen to one extent or another.

This is very much like high trapeze artists who may be extremely skilled and fly from one trapeze to another like birds. The odds of their missing their hold and falling is rare, but if they fall and there is no safety net, they will get hurt or die.

Also, if they are still under training or if they are established players but simply out of shape or fatigued, the odds of falling are higher and without a safety net the risk of hurting or killing themselves is significantly higher.

It is this concept of a safety net that prompted me in 1989 to try and develop a technique and/or a machine that would have some sort of inherent safety mechanism independent of the surgeon's level of skill so that if the active tip accidently touches the capsule or iris or any other structure of the anterior segment, little or no damage happens.

I started by outlining for myself the different mechanisms by which the posterior capsule can be ruptured during phacoemulsification. The actual mechanisms by which the posterior capsule could be ruptured are basically one of the following:

- Extension around the equator of a break in the continuous tear anterior capsulorhexis.

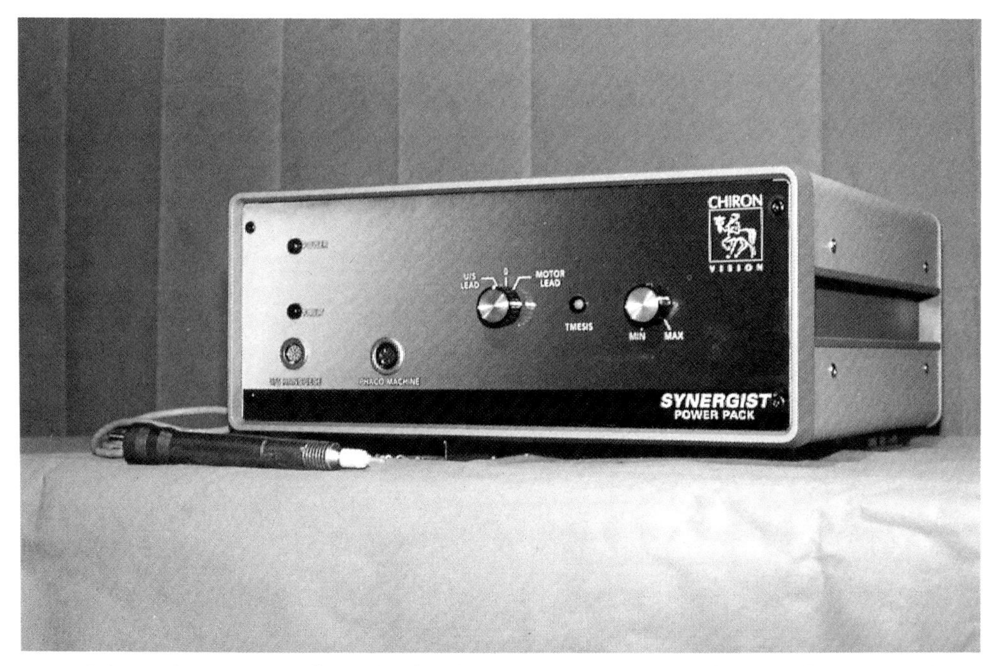

Figure 8-2. The Chiron Tmesis Synergist. Can be made to work with any phaco machine to provide Tmesis.

- Posterior capsular contact with the point or the sharp side of the bevel on the ultrasonically active tip. This can occur due to a sudden inadvertent movement of the tip, or due to a sudden decrease in anterior chamber pressure causing forward movement of the posterior capsule.
- Posterior capsular capture and rupture by occlusion of the port of the moving, actively aspirating, ultrasonic phaco tip. Moreover, it is obvious that the phacoemulsification tip acts as a vibrating chisel pointing directly toward the posterior capsule.

In analyzing all current phacoemulsification techniques it becomes immediately evident that no matter how different each technique claims to be, and no matter which machine is used or what ultrasound, flow rate, and vacuum parameters (Table 8-1) are preferred, there are two basic stages or steps common to all of them:

- Reduction of the nucleus into small fragments.
- Ultrasonic aspiration of the nuclear fragments.

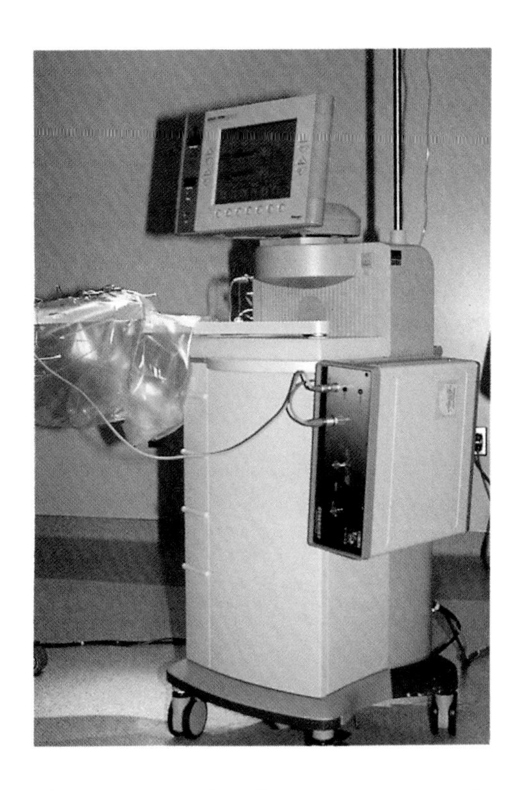

Figure 8-3. Chiron Tmesis Synergist connected to the Alcon LEGACY machine.

It is during this second stage or step of the operation that the posterior capsule becomes most vulnerable to damage. As the nuclear fragments are gradually removed, more and more of the posterior capsule becomes completely exposed or covered by a thin layer of nonprotective cortical fibers. This is the time when any inadvertent contact between the posterior capsule and the active phaco tip would almost invariably lead to rupture of the posterior capsule and invasion of the operative field with uncooperative, intrusive, and sticky vitreous, leading to less than optimal final surgical outcomes for the patient and disappointment for the surgeon.

History, Development, and Evolution

My objective in the development and evolution of Tmesis (Table 8-2) was to develop an inherent safety mechanism in the instrument itself. My thoughts were to somehow find a way of making the instrument differentiate between the structurally friable nuclear particles and the smooth capsular membrane, attacking the former and protecting the latter.

My initial idea was to use a ring that rotates at high speeds around its diameter. It would connect with an aspirating cannula in line with its diameter. Its advancing edges as it rotates would be sharp and its receding edges blunt. The way it worked was as it rapidly rotates it would form a hollow sphere that opened into the aspirating cannula. When brought into contact with the nucleus, it would shave slivers from the nucleus in a tangential direction (hence the term "Tmesis," Greek for cutting) and these slivers within the hollow sphere would be immediately aspirated through the aspiration cannula. Moreover, the receding edge would leave a trail of cavitation leading to further collapse of the nuclear matter.

However, when this rotating sphere would come in contact with the capsule, which is a membranous structure with a smooth surface, it would glide along its surface causing it no harm.

The prototype of this model certainly did work and did differentiate between nuclear matter and membranous capsule, however, the tissue removal effect was not efficient enough to be practical. Moreover, the rotating ring presented a closed surface at its distal end which further impeded nuclear tissue removal.

To enhance the nuclear tissue removal effect I decided to add ultrasound energy simultaneously with rotation. This was no easy technological feat for Mark Steen, the engineer of this project, who is also my friend and partner in PhacoTmesis. Nevertheless, he did succeed in designing and producing a handpiece that provided simultaneous ultrasonic linear oscillation and high speed rotation (Tables 8-3 and 8-4).

To overcome the problem with the closed front end of the ring, the tip was changed to a cannula split at its distal end with the two halves slightly offset. This configuration improved the tissue removal significantly. However, at that stage of evolution of Tmesis, I was under the wrong impression that the technique for Tmesis would utilize the powerful tissue ablative effect at the tip to attack the intact nucleus from the center outwards until the nucleus is all removed. In order to do this the Tmesis tip had to be extended beyond the irrigation sleeve as much as the phaco tip and therefore exposed the capsule to the same risk of damage as phaco would, particularly if a sharp Tmesis tip was used.

Moreover, the slits on the sides of the cannula prevented occludability and thus slowed down the procedure. At first the slits were thought to enhance the effectiveness of the tip in nuclear tissue removal, however, surgical experience with non-slitted tips proved them to be more efficient.

I, therefore, had to rethink my approach, and return to current strategies in phacoemulsification, that is:

- Reduce the whole nucleus down to fragments.
- Aspirate the nuclear fragments.

Once I started following this strategy, the unique features of Tmesis (Table 8-5) instantly crystallized and I realized that now, finally, I have accomplished the objective that has eluded me for more than 5 years.

This objective, this unique feature is:

- When the Tmesis tip is properly assembled with the irrigating silicone sleeve completely covering the ultrasonically active, rotating Tmesis tip (Figure 8-4), it is capable of removing the nuclear fragments (Figure 8-5) with superior efficiency.
- If at any time during this stage of nuclear removal the posterior capsule or the iris comes in contact with the instrument it will not be damaged. This inherent safety feature could not be duplicated by any existing phaco machine. It should be clearly obvious that there is no mystery in this safety feature. There simply is no sharp, beveled or non-beveled oscillating or rotating tip exposed to touch any vital tissue and cause harm. The reasons, however, that it is so effective in removing the nuclear fragments are:
    1. The combined ultrasonic oscillation and high speed rotation create a pulverizing effect on the friable nuclear fragments at a slight distance from the tip. That is, actual contact with the tip is not necessary.
    2. The rotation at the Tmesis tip causes a circular fluid current in the direction of rotation. This combined with the aspiration flow creates a mini whirlpool that keeps the followability of the nuclear fragments into the pulverizing aspiration zone.

The Tmesis tips come in 0.6 mm and 0.9 mm caliber. I personally prefer the 0.6 mm because I like to operate intercapsularly. We used to have a teflon irrigation sleeve; I did not like it because it offers more resistance when moving at the incision site and friction with the iris stroma superiorly can cause some partial loss of that tissue.

The new transparent silicone sleeve is a joy to work with. Its advantages are:

- Its transparency makes the Tmesis tip within visible and helps proper adjustment of its position to overlap the distal end of the Tmesis tip.
- It glides into the incision very easily and therefore movement of the instrument does not move the whole eye.

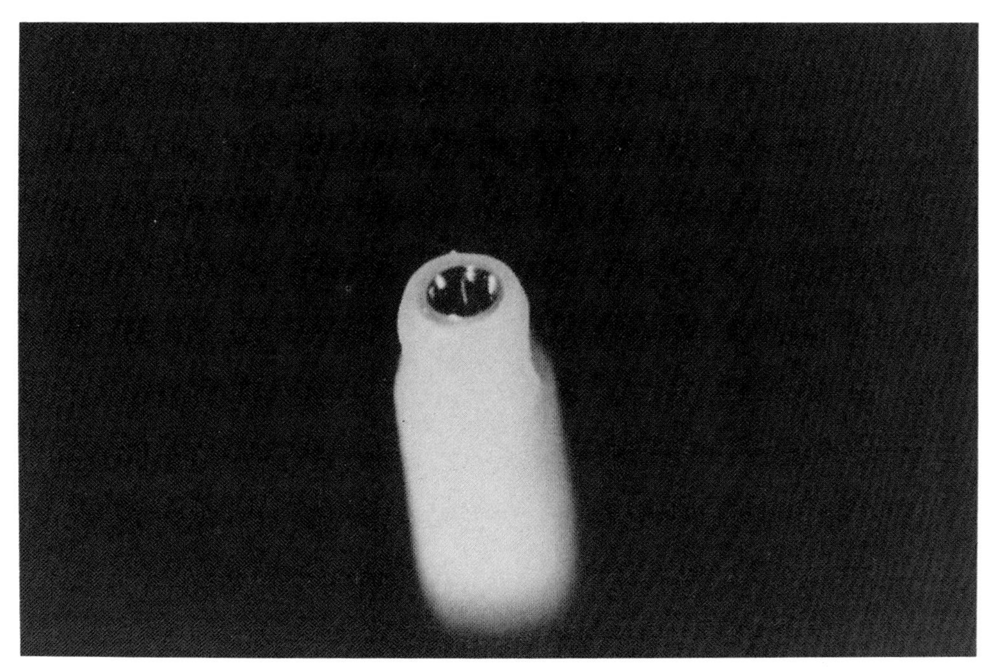

Figure 8-4. Tmesis tip in active mode. The irrigating sleeve covers active tip completely and overlaps it.

- It does not damage the incision or the iris.
- It conforms better to the incision preventing fluid leakage from the anterior chamber thus offering better maintenance of its depth.

Tmesis Procedure

To perform PhacoTmesis, the surgeon does not have to learn a new technique or convert from his or her current favorite technique of phacoemulsification in which a high level of skill and confidence has been acquired. Any current technique of phacoemulsification can be performed with Tmesis with equal, if not more, efficiency and speed with the added advantage of the inherent safety to the posterior capsule and iris.

The following is an outline of the procedural steps to perform each of the these major techniques of phacoemulsification and their variations using Tmesis:

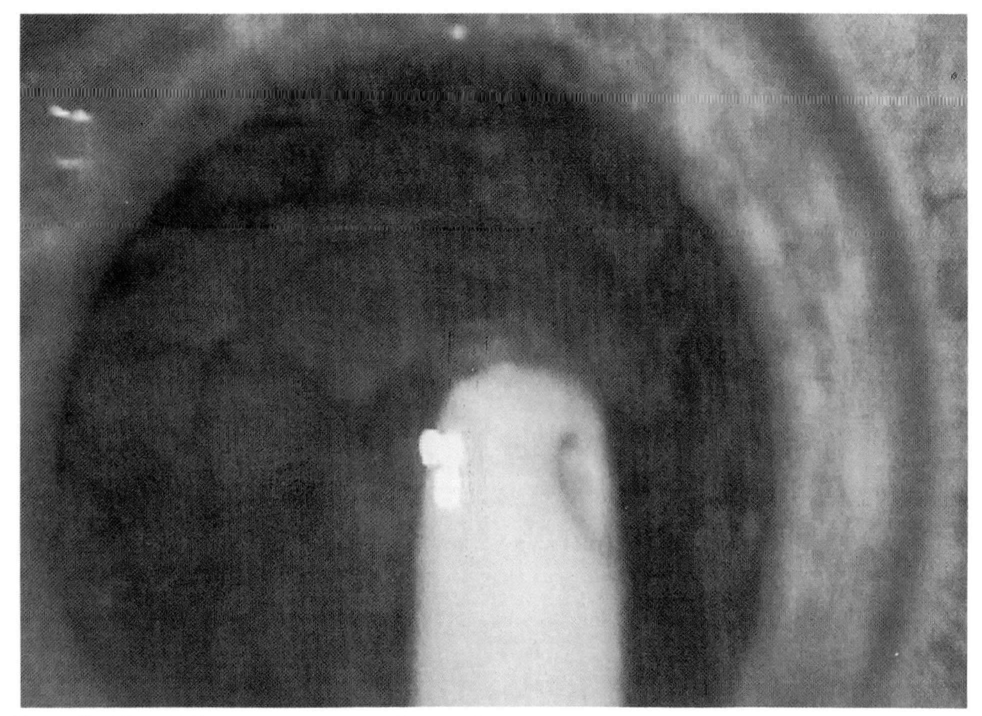

Figure 8-5. Tmesis tip removing nuclear fragments.

I. Divide and Conquer Techniques

A. Incision
   1. Surgeon's preference
B. Anterior capsulorhexis
   1. Surgeon's preference
C. Hydrodissection and hydrodelineation
   1. Surgeon's preference
D. Nuclear division
   1. Tmesis tip extended out of irrigating sleeve to surgeon's preference
   2. Mode: Simultaneous ultrasound and rotation
   3. Settings:
      a. Ultrasound: 50% to 60% or surgeon's preference
      b. Rotation: 5000 to 7000 rpm
   4. Flow rate: surgeon's preference
   5. Vacuum: surgeon's preference

E. Tmesis of nuclear fragments
   1. Tmesis tip withdrawn completely within irrigating sleeve
   2. Mode: simultaneous ultrasound and rotation
   3. Settings: U/S 50% to 60%
   4. Flow rate: 20 mL/min
   5. Vacuum: 60 to 120 mmHg
F. Residual cortical removal
   1. Tmesis tip: same as above
   2. Mode: aspiration and irrigation
   3. Settings: same as above or surgeon's preference

II. Phaco Chop Techniques

A. Incision
   1. Surgeon's preference
B. Anterior capsulorhexis
   1. Surgeon's preference
C. Hydrodissection and hydrodelineation
   1. Surgeon's preference
D. Nuclear chopping
   1. Tmesis tip extended out of irrigating sleeve to surgeon's preference
   2. Mode: ultrasound only
   3. Settings:
      a. Ultrasound: 50% to 60% or surgeon's preference
      b. Flow rate: surgeon's preference
      c. Vacuum: 150 to 200 mmHg or surgeon's preference
E. Tmesis of nuclear fragments
   1. Same as in divide and conquer
F. Residual cortex removal
   1. Same as in divide and conquer

III. Hydrosonic Intercapsular "HIT" Tmesis Technique

A. Incision
   1. Surgeon's preference
B. Anterior capsulorhexis
   1. 2 to 3 mm in diameter
   2. Just within pupillary border in line with incision
C. Hydrodissection
   1. Hydrosonic cannula and handpiece (new Alcon-enhanced hydrosonics Handpiece Legacy)
D. Hydrodelineation and hydrofragmentation of nuclear core and epinucleus (Figure 8-6)
   1. Position 3 on foot control
   2. Ultrasound power 50% to 90%
   3. Pulse frequency setting position 4
E. Tmesis of nuclear fragments
   1. Tmesis tip withdrawn completely within irrigating sleeve
   2. Mode: simultaneous ultrasound and rotation
   3. Settings:
      a. Ultrasound: 50% to 60%
      b. Flow rate: 20 mL/min (continuous flow)
      c. Vacuum: 60 to 120 mmHg
   4. Single instrument technique
F. Residual cortex removal
   1. Same as previous techniques

IV. Hydrosonic Endocapsular "HET" Tmesis Technique

Same as "HIT" Technique except for the following:

A. Anterior capsulorhexis' central large about 6 mm in diameter
B. Surgeon is free to use single instrument technique or add a nuclear manipulator to manipulate the nuclear fragments through a paracentesis incision.

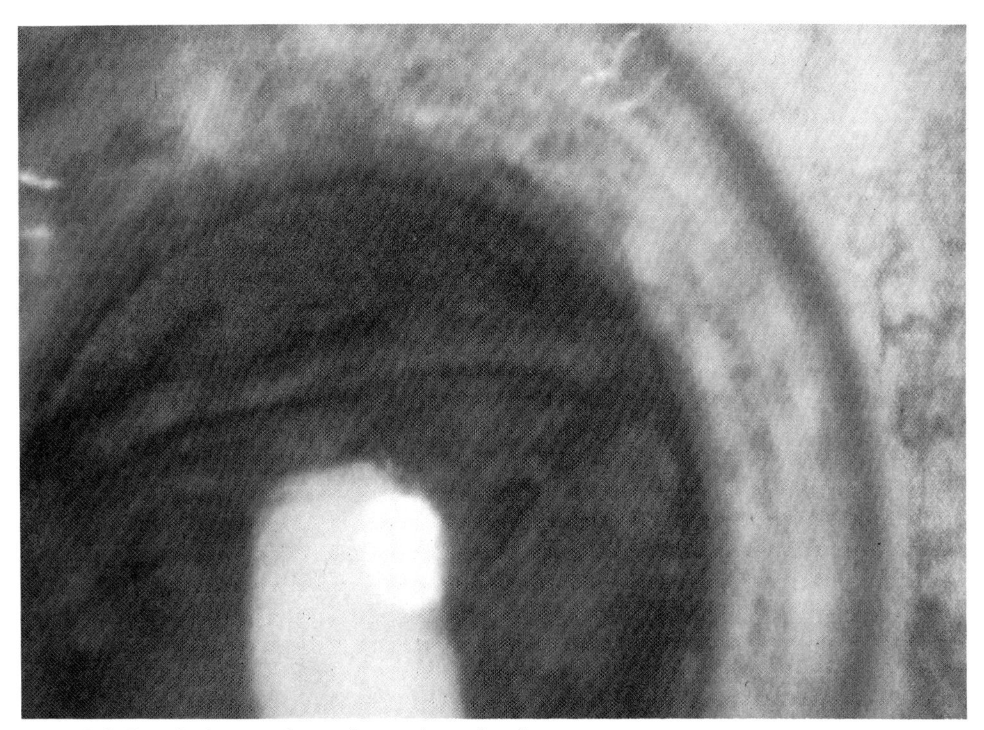

Figure 8-6. Tmesis tip engaging and removing epinucleus.

Table 8-1. Tmesis Procedure: Chiron Synergist Attached to Alcon LEGACY 20000

Tmesis Tip small diameter, zero degree bevel, silicone sleeve		
Power		50%
Aspiration		20/cc
Vacuum		60 to 120 mmHg
Mode		Linear
Hydrosonics		
Pressure		60 ppm
Power		60%
Rate		5

Table 8-2. Tmesis Cataract Extraction System

Mission:
A full-featured anterior segment system that gives the surgeon state-of-the-art technology.

- Breakthrough technology multifunction handpiece
- New family of ultrasonic handpieces
- Binary fluidics for safe, effective peristaltic pump action
- Full programmability of surgical parameters to memory key system
- Simplified user interface for rapid changeover

Table 8-3. Chiron Vision Tmesis Multifunction Handpiece: Features and Benefits

Simultaneous ultrasonic stroke and high-speed rotation	Associated energies fragment and mill nuclear material into a fine mix. Extremely important in small-incision surgery. Rotational energies create "Microsphere Fluidics" that appear to be capsule friendly. Rotational settings are programmable up to 10,000 rpm.
Powerful 4 mil ultrasonic stroke	Rotation/ultrasound combination can handle the hardest nucleus.
Zero degree bevel ultrasonic tip	Non-beveled tip enhances capsule-friendly environment.
Foot switch activation	Allows surgeon the flexibility to turn rotation on or off as the procedure progresses.

Table 8-4. Chiron Vision Magnum Ultrasonic Handpiece: Features and Benefits

All-titanium construction	Lightweight and durable. Easy to maneuver. Less hand fatigue.
Autosense tuning	Smooth, consistent stroke that adjusts for changing nuclear densities.
Coaxial infusion system	Eliminates external tubing for easier maneuverability.
Reduced length	Shorter length is ideal for temporal approach. Less chance of restricted movement.

Table 8-5. Chiron Vision Tmesis Cataract Extraction System: Features and Benefits

Feature	Benefit
High efficiency Binary Fluidics system	Safety of peristaltic, response of "vacuum on demand."
Unique autoload tubing set-up (AVPC)	Simple and quick set-up. Ensures proper loading of pump tubing.
Automated set-up of ultrasonics and fluidics	Quickly verifies correct operation of vacuum and ultrasonics.
Full-time "manual mode" with safety of presets	Instantly adjust vacuum, aspiration, panel/surgeon control, power, constant irrigation, cutting, and all other functions.
Easy and total programmability	Quick set-up for OR with multiple surgeons or multiple techniques for one surgeon.
Remote site diagnostics (CIA)	Remote link-up to troubleshoot, minor recalibration, and monitor performance.
Sterile field remote control	Full access to all intraoperative adjustments from the sterile field.
True linear vacuum	Up-down control of vacuum. Safety of peristaltic, response of vacuum on demand.
Preset capsule vacuum mode	Low aspiration and vacuum settings, reduces delays in OR.
Adjustable vit cutting rate	Offers flexibility for surgeon's preference.
Full-line vit cutters	Offers flexibility for surgeon's preference.
Built-in coagulation	Less clutter in the OR. One foot switch.
Programmable audible tones	Customize for surgeon's requirements.
Adjustable volume control	Customize for surgeon's requirements.
Vacuum units programmable	Customize for surgeon's preference.
All surgical parameters can be memorized, intuitive operation	Quick to learn, easy to remember.
One key, one function	Minimizes confusion.

Chapter 9

Current Techniques in Laser Cataract Surgery

Jack M. Dodick, MD
Laurence T. D. Sperber, MD

In the other chapters in this book, we have learned a great deal of information about ultrasound phacoemulsification. Ultrasound phacoemulsification has come a long way since its creation by Dr. Charles Kelman.[1] The first phacoemulsification procedure took over 3 hours and used more than an hour of phacoemulsification time (Dr. Charles Kelman, personal communication). Now, after years of improvements and refinements, ultrasound phacoemulsification has revolutionized cataract surgery and currently defines small-incision cataract surgery as removing a lens through a 3.2-mm or smaller incision.

Despite the continuing refinements and improvements in ultrasound phacoemulsification, which have resulted in its increasing popularity, ultrasound phacoemulsification is not a perfect procedure. Many surgeons find the bulky handpiece ergonometrically uncomfortable and, therefore, somewhat difficult to use. In addition, the learning curve is a steep one, and because of this, many surgeons who have been performing primarily planned extracapsular cataract extraction find converting to phacoemulsification a hazardous and uncomfortable proposition. Also, because ultrasound energy is released beyond the tip of the phacoemulsification probe, there is the potential of injuring the corneal endothelium, posterior capsule, and iris. Because of the presence of a piezo-electric crystal in the handpiece, the handpiece is subject to frequent breakdown. It would be a significant improvement, therefore, to create an instrument capable of cataract removal which utilizes a smaller, safer, and more reliable handpiece.

For the above reasons, as well as the desire to improve upon the cataract operation, investigators have, over the last few years, been searching for alternative energy sources to ultrasound for cataract removal. In this chapter, we focus on laser energy as such an alternative energy source. The wavelengths currently under investigation for cataract removal include: Nd:YAG 1064 nm,[2-4] Nd:YLF 1053 nm,[5] Er:YAG 2940 nm,[6-8] and four ultraviolet (excimer) laser wavelengths—193 nm (argon fluoride), 248 nm (krypton fluoride), 308 nm (xenon chloride), and 351 nm (xenon fluoride).[9-17]

While excimer laser is clearly the future of keratorefractive surgery, its use in devices capable of cataract removal has not been as promising. The four wavelengths of excimer laser energy which have been studied for cataract removal are 193 nm, 248 nm, 308 nm, and 351 nm. However, 351 nm was found to be ineffective in cataract ablation, so ongoing research has focused on the remaining three wavelengths.[9-17]

In a study by Puliafito et al[16] human cadaver and bovine lenses were treated with both 193 nm and 248 nm excimer laser energy. These treatments resulted in perforation of the lens capsule and the creation of smooth-walled ablation zones. Examination of these lenses with light microscopy, transmission, and scanning electron microscopy revealed smooth ablation zones without any adjacent charring of the lens tissue. While 248 nm excimer energy ablated the cornea at lower levels of energy, ablation with 193 nm excimer energy was more precise. Smooth-walled incisions were made with the 193 nm excimer, while 248 nm excimer created more jagged appearing incisions. The incisions created by 248 nm excimer were also surrounded by an adjacent stromal damage zone of more than 2.5 microns in width.[15,16]

Nanevicz et al[13] performed a study examining the effects of 193 nm, 248 nm, 308 nm, and 351 nm excimer laser energy on the bovine crystalline lens. Absorbance, rate, precision, and threshold of were studied. The study revealed that 351 nm laser energy did not prove capable of ablation. Also noted, 248 nm had the highest rate of ablation, but it was also the least precise. With regard to all of the study parameters, 193 nm appeared to be the wavelength of choice for cataract removal. However, given the current limits of fiber optic technology, transmission of 193 nm excimer laser energy through a fiber optic is currently not feasible.[13]

The Nanevicz et al[13] study demonstrated that 308 nm is the best wavelength overall for cataract removal. It has a higher ablation threshold than 193 nm, but it is more precise in its ablation than 248 nm. In addition, 308 nm excimer laser energy can be transmitted through a fiber optic. Also, it has been theorized that 308 nm energy stimulates a photochemical reaction, promoting ablation by producing UV-absorbing chromophores.[10,11,13]

Maguen et al[10] examined 308 nm excimer laser energy delivered through a fiber optic and its effects on the human cadaver lens. They found that the ablation threshold of the lens capsule, both anterior and posterior, was significantly higher than that of both the nucleus and cortex. This higher ablation threshold suggests that 308 nm excimer laser transmitted by a fiber optic system is a potentially safe energy source for use in cataract removal.[10]

Despite all of the research into the various excimer wavelengths, and the creation of several workable devices using 308 nm excimer laser energy to remove cataracts, the FDA has not approved any of them for human clinical trials.[9-17] The most likely reasons why FDA approval has not occurred are the possibility of retinal toxicity and carcinogenesis from exposure to excimer laser energy,[11,18-20] as well as the fact that ultraviolet radiation of 308 nm has been shown to be cataractogenic in humans.[11,19,21] It is unlikely that the FDA will approve any intraocular device that utilizes 308 nm excimer laser energy for human clinical trials until further study of these effects can be completed. Also, additional shielding, protecting both the eyes of the surgeon and the surrounding structures of the patient's eye, will have to be incorporated into the existing devices before the FDA will consider its approval.

Because of the safety concerns with the ultraviolet wavelengths, a great deal of attention has been focused on the infrared wavelengths as an energy source for cataract removal. At the American Society of Cataract and Refractive Surgery Annual Meeting in March 1990, Dr. Stuart Brown first presented his work on the Nd:YLF 1053 nm picosecond laser.[5] Since that time, several investigators have demonstrated that the 1053 nm picosecond laser is capable of both corneal and lens ablation. Intrastromal corneal ablation using this laser has shown great potential for refractive surgery, as it can reshape the central cornea without damage to Bowman's layer.[5] Dr. Brown and his co-workers report that the 1053 nm picosecond laser can be used to treat human cataracts in a fashion similar to the way the Nd:YAG laser has been used for photophacofragmentation, but with greater precision.[5] The laser energy softens the lens nucleus and cortex. After the laser treatment is completed, the treated lens material can be removed using a standard irrigation/aspiration probe and, if necessary, ultrasound phacoemulsification. The goal of this treatment is to reduce or eliminate the need for ultrasound phacoemulsification.

A human clinical trial was completed in which the posterior half of the cataractous human lens was treated with laser while the anterior half was left untreated. In all the patients, the need for ultrasound phacoemulsification energy was completely eliminated. That is, the treated half of the lens was removed using an irrigation/aspiration probe alone. The untreated half of the lens required the use of ultrasound phacoemulsification for its removal. This procedure is very controlled and uses very low energy; consequently, there have been no reported intraocular pressure rises prior to doing the phacoemulsification procedure (Dr. David Schanzlin, personal communication). Further studies are underway. The most significant disadvantage of this procedure is the fact that it is a two-staged procedure, and to date, no intraocular device using this wavelength has been developed.

Another infrared laser wavelength, Erbium:YAG (2.94 nm), is also being investigated for the removal of cataracts. Drs. Peyman and Katoh have utilized three different systems for the delivering Er:YAG laser energy: an aluminum mask, an iris diaphragm, and a 150 micron fiber optic fiber. These different delivery systems were used to ablate the lens, make a corneal incision, perform an iridotomy, and make a retinal incision. The tissue was examined after the laser treatments using scanning electron and light microscopy. These examinations revealed a picture was similar to the photoablation of the lens and cornea produced by the excimer laser. Adjacent to these ablated areas, there was a very narrow zone of surrounding thermal effect.[7]

In his study using pulsed Er:YAG laser energy transmitted through a 400 micron fiber optic probe, Tsubota treated the cornea, trabecular meshwork, lens, and vitreous of enucleated rabbit eyes. After laser treatment, the tissue was studied by both light and scanning electron microscopy. At low energy levels, coagulation of the cornea and lens was seen, while at higher energy levels, ablation was observed. The area adjacent to the ablation zone was covered with a powdery substance which Dr. Tsubota felt was ablated tissue. Thermal effects were also seen in this region.[8]

Premier Laser Systems and Dr. D. Michael Colvard have developed an Erbium:YAG laser device for the removal of cataracts. The device is a probe with an olive-tipped, fluoride-based fiber. A fluoride-based material was used because Er:YAG laser energy is highly absorbed by water, and other fiber materials, such as quartz, have a higher water content. This device has been used to perform a capsulotomy with the same properties and appearance as a continuous curvilinear capsulorhexis, in that its continuous edge is quite strong and resists radial tearing. After the capsulotomy, the olive-tipped fiber is passed over the surface of the nucleus like an eraser, and this ablates the cataractous lens. The ablated material is aspirated out of the eye using an aspiration system. To date, the laser probe has been used to remove the anterior portion of the nucleus and then a standard ultrasound phacoemulsification probe has been used to remove the rest of the nucleus[6] (Dr. D. Michael Colvard, personal communication).

In animal studies, no significant damage to corneal endothelium or other intraocular structures has been seen. Premarket Approval (PMA) for performing anterior capsulotomy has been granted by the FDA, as well as an Investigational Device Exemption (IDE) for cataract ablation and for sclerotomy[6] (Dr. D. Michael Colvard, personal communication). Under an IDE, more than 20 cases with the Er:YAG Laser have been performed by Dr. Colvard and his co-investigators. Dr. Colvard reports that these cases, combining the laser with standard ultrasound phacoemulsification, have been very successful, with the patients doing very well. While it is still relatively early in its development, with further adjustments to the probe necessary, this technology appears to be on the right track to becoming an alternative to ultrasound phacoemulsification (Dr. D. Michael Colvard, personal communication).

In contrast to ultraviolet lasers, there have been no reports of retinal toxicity or mutagenesis (seen with ultraviolet radiation) with Er:YAG.[18,20] Therefore, Er:YAG appears to be safer than ultraviolet energy. In addition, because it is possible to transmit Er:YAG laser through a fiber optic fiber, there is great potential for use in cataract extraction and other intraocular surgery.

Another relatively new infrared laser has been developed by Dr. Daniel Eichenbaum in conjunction with a company named Paradigm Medical Industries. It utilizes a solid-state pulsed Nd:YAG laser which delivers the laser energy to the cataract through a fiber optic into a probe which has irrigation and aspiration connected to it. The cataract is disrupted when it comes in contact with the laser energy within the probe. The company has just recently been granted an IDE by the FDA and clinical trials should begin in the near future. Once underway, clinical data regarding the safety and efficacy of this probe should be available, but to date, there have been no published reports in peer-reviewed ophthalmology journals on this technology.[22]

When examining the laser devices discussed in this article so far, there is a common mechanism of action they all possess: the cataract is removed by applying the laser energy directly to the cataract. This approach has led to several effective laser devices, however, the drawback with this approach is that there is direct exposure of both the eyes of the patient and the surgeon to laser light. With the excimer laser devices, this has raised safety concerns.[18-21] I (JMD) have developed a laser-driven device that does not utilize the direct effects of the laser source to disrupt the patient's cataract. Instead, shock waves created by a Nd:YAG laser striking a titanium target disrupt the lens. This approach shields both the eyes of the patient and the surgeon from exposure to the Nd:YAG laser energy.[2]

In October 1989, I (JMD) first presented my Laser Lens Ablation device at the American Academy of Ophthalmology Annual Meeting. The energy source for this device is a pulsed Nd:YAG 1064 nm laser transmitted through a fiber optic to a probe. The probe houses a 300 micron quartz clad fiber optic fiber which terminates approximately 1 mm in front of a titanium target. This target is adjacent to the mouth of the probe. The proximal end of the quartz fiber is connected to the laser source by a standard laser connector. This target is the key element of this device.[2,3]

The pulsed laser energy, delivered by the quartz fiber, strikes the titanium target which causes optical breakdown and plasma formation to occur. Because titanium greatly reduces the threshold for optical breakdown and plasma formation, this phenomenon can occur at very low energy, as compared to the very high energy required without a target. The resultant optical breakdown causes shock waves to emanate toward the distal opening of the probe. It is at this opening where the shock waves come in contact with the lens material which is held in approximation with the tip of the probe by the suction created by the aspiration port. The shock waves disrupt the cataract, and the particles of lens material are aspirated out of the eye. In simplest terms, the target acts as a transducer, converting laser energy into shock waves which ablate the nucleus. In addition to functioning as a transducer, the target shields the surrounding tissues of the patient's eye, namely the corneal endothelium, iris, posterior capsule, and retina of the patient, as well as the eyes of the surgeon, from direct laser light.[2,3]

Once the initial studies proved that Laser Lens Ablation was capable of ablating the cataractous human cadaver lens,[2] we performed the first animal study in order to assess the safety of Laser Lens Ablation. The laser probe was inserted into the anterior chamber of one eye of 15 New Zealand white rabbits and the laser energy was discharged, exposing the rabbit eyes to a level of laser energy which was significantly greater than that required to ablate the cataractous cadaver lens as determined in previous in vitro studies. The procedure was done in one eye per rabbit, with the fellow, non-operated eye serving as a control. After the procedures were performed, the rabbits were sacrificed and both eyes were enucleated at three postoperative times (1 hour, 1 day, and 1 week). The eyes were examined by specular microscopy, ultrasonic pachymetry, and light microscopy, and no damage to the corneal endothelium, trabecular meshwork, or retina of the rabbit eye was seen.[22,23]

Further refinement of the laser probe was done with the aid of a method of high speed photography developed by Christiansen and myself (JMD) which allowed the investigators to study the formation and propagation of shock waves created after the Nd:YAG laser pulses strike the titanium target of the Dodick Laser Lens Ablation device. As this method of high speed photography has provided me and my co-workers a great deal of information regarding the production and propagation of the shock waves produced by the laser device, the target and laser probe configuration have been modified to produce the safest, most efficient, and most effective device. These studies have resulted in a much safer and more efficient probe, allowing for far less input laser energy to be used in the ablation of cataracts. The ultimate goal of these modifications is to produce a probe with the maximum shock wave output up to but not beyond the mouth of the probe, which allows for the most efficient use of the laser energy and prevents its escape, thus making a safer, more effective probe.[4]

I (JMD) have been performing Nd:YAG Laser Lens Ablation under an IDE from the FDA since July 1991, when the first human case was performed. These procedures have been performed using a surgical technique which is virtually identical to one-handed endocapsular phacoemulsification, except of course, that the laser probe is used. Minimal postoperative inflammation and endothelial cell loss have been encountered. The first patient has been followed for more than 3 years and continues to do well, maintaining a postoperative visual acuity of 20/40 which was equivalent to the preoperative Potential Acuity Meter (PAM) measurement.[3]

In the time since the first case, significant improvements have been made. These changes have made the laser device more efficient, allowing the probe to be used with the same technique as the first case but with much less Nd:YAG laser energy required. Because of the similarity to ultrasound phacoemulsification, the procedure should be easily mastered by the accomplished phacoemulsification surgeon. Because the probe is smaller and ergonomically more comfortable than the ultrasound phacoemulsification handpiece, extracapsular cataract surgeons and novice phacoemulsification surgeons should be able to perform this procedure comfortably.

To date, a total of 11 patients have had their cataracts removed with the Laser Lens Ablation device and all of the patients have had excellent results with no adverse effects seen in follow-up.

Since the advent of ultrasound phacoemulsification, we have witnessed an incredible evolution in cataract surgery. The progression from intracapsular cataract extraction to planned extracapsular cataract extraction to ultrasound phacoemulsification has improved the results of cataract surgery by leaps and bounds, making it a safer and easier procedure, both for the patient and for the surgeon. Over the past few years, the search for alternative methods of cataract removal has led investigators to attempt to harness laser energy in the removal of cataracts. At present, there are several devices capable of cataract removal. Human clinical trials of two devices are underway and the results to date have been excellent to date; in addition, a clinical trial of a third device will commence shortly. Given the interest and the ongoing research, as well as the experimental results and the number of different laser systems being studied, it is clear that the dream of laser cataract surgery is rapidly approaching reality. This dream is fostered by a desire to create and produce a safer and more effective device to perform small-incision cataract surgery.

References

1. Kelman CD. Phaco-emulsification and aspiration: a new technique of cataract removal. A preliminary report. *Am J Ophthalmol.* 1967;64(1):23-35.
2. Dodick JM. Laser phacolysis of the human cataractous lens. *Dev Ophthalmol* (Basil, Switzerland). 1991;22:58-64.
3. Dodick JM, Sperber LTD, Lally JM, Kazlas M. Laser phacolysis of the human cataractous lens. *Arch Ophthalmol.* 1993;111:903-904.
4. Dodick JM, Christiansen J. Experimental studies on the development and propagation of shock waves created by the interaction of short Nd:YAG laser pulses with a titanium target: possible implications for Nd:YAG laser phacolysis of the cataractous human lens. *J Cataract Refract Surg.* 1991;17(6):794-797.
5. Brown S. The multipurpose 1053 picosecond laser. Presented to the American Society of Cataract and Refractive Surgery (ASCRS) Annual Meeting; March 1990.
6. Colvard DM. Erbium:YAG laser removal of cataracts. Presented to the American Academy of Ophthalmology Annual Meeting; November 1994; San Francisco, Calif.
7. Peyman GA, Katoh N. Effects of an erbium:YAG laser on ocular structures. *Int Ophthalmol.* 1987;10:245-253.
8. Tsubota K. Application of erbium:YAG laser in ocular ablation. *Ophthalmologica.* 1990;200(3):117-122.
9. Bath PE, Kar H, Apple DJ, et al. Endocapsular excimer laser phakoablation through a 1-mm incision. *Ophthalmic Laser Therapy.* 1987;2(4):245-248.
10. Maguen E, Martinez M, Grundfest W, et al. Excimer laser ablation of the human lens at 308 nm with a fiber delivery system. *J Cataract Refract Surg. 1989;15:409-414.*
11. Marshall J, Sliney DH. Endoexcimer laser intraocular ablative photodecomposition. *Am J Ophthalmol.* 1986;101(1):130-131. Letter.
12. Muller-Stolzenburg N, Muller GJ. Transmission of 308 nm excimer laser radiation for ophthalmic microsurgery—medical, technical and safety aspects. *Biomed Tech* (Berlin). 1989;34(6):131-138.
13. Nanevicz T, Prince MR, Gawande AA, et al. Excimer laser ablation of the lens. *Arch Ophthalmol.* 1986;104:1825-1829.
14. Pellin MJ, Williams GA, Young CE, et al. Endoexcimer laser intraocular ablative photodecomposition. *Am J Ophthalmol.* 1985;99(4):483-484. Letter.
15. Puliafito CA, Steinert RF. Laser surgery of the lens: experimental studies. *Ophthalmology.* 1983;90(8):1007-1012.
16. Puliafito CA, Steinert RF, Deutsch TF, et al. Excimer laser ablation of the cornea and lens: experimental studies. *Ophthalmology.* 1985;92:741-748.
17. Peyman GA, Kuszak JR, Weckstrom K, et al. Effects of XeCl excimer laser on the eye-

lid and anterior segment structures. *Arch Ophthalmol.* 1986;104:118-122.

18. Kochevar IE. Cytotoxicity and mutagenicity of excimer laser radiation. *Lasers Surg Med.* 1989;9(5):440-445.
19. Zuclich JA. Ultraviolet-induced photochemical damage in ocular tissues. *Health Physics.* 1989;56(5):671-682.
20. Trentacoste J, Thompson K, Parrish II RK, et al. Mutagenic potential of a 193 nm excimer laser on fibroblasts in tissue culture. *Ophthalmology.* 1987; 94:125-129.
21. Borkman RF. Cataracts and photochemical damage in the lens. *Ciba Found Symp.* 1984;106:88-109.
22. Kronemyer B. First computer-aided, laser cataract removal system ready for clinical trials. *Ocular Surgery News.* May 1, 1995.
23. Sperber LTD, Dodick JM. Nd:YAG laser phacolysis: an acute study in rabbits. In press.

Chapter 10

Paradigm System: A Laser Probe for Cataract Removal

Daniel M. Eichenbaum, MD

The first decade of ultrasonic phacoemulsification cannot be considered an overwhelming success in terms of physician acceptance. Use of the equipment and technique was limited to a handful of surgeons who mastered the difficult operation by persevering through the long and arduous learning curve. Implant technology and design lagged well behind surgical technique to the point that implants designed for intracapsular surgery were being inserted through small phacoemulsification incisions enlarged to 8 mm or more.

One principle that emerged from the chaos, however, was that an intact posterior capsule did in fact protect the eye from complications such as retinal detachment and cystoid macular edema. Additionally, a shorter incision proved to be more stable and more predictable in terms of postoperative astigmatism and patient activity. Finally, with the development of the posterior chamber implant, a decrease in implant-related complications was achieved.

In the early 1980s, therefore, ophthalmic surgeons were being dragged, sometimes with great pain for all concerned, into the modern era of extracapsular cataract extraction with posterior chamber lens implantation. Many surgeons tried ultrasonic phacoemulsification, but most chose to perform extracapsular surgery with expression of the intact nucleus and to use some form of irrigation/aspiration device for cortical clean-up. The planned extracapsular technique did not involve holding a vibrating needle inside the confines of the anterior chamber. That vibrating needle would shred any tissue it contacted (iris, posterior capsule, cornea, etc). Mastering an irrigation/aspiration probe for cortex removal was a much easier task. The necessity of enlarging the incision for the implant was further justification for eschewing ultrasonics for a simpler and, in the hands of most, safer technique.

In 1983, with the status of cataract surgery as outlined above, I began the process of developing the laser probe for intraocular tissue removal. My primary goal was to develop a device that was completely user-friendly to the average surgeon, a probe as familiar and easy to use as the irrigation/aspiration needle. The choice of the Nd:YAG wavelength was based on theory (from absorption graphs) and availability of the laser. An initial feasibility study was designed and performed using human cataract nuclei removed from patients undergoing planned extracapsular cataract surgery. Optical fiber technology at that time was geared primarily toward light transmission for communications applications. Power transmission fiber technology was poorly developed. The objectives, therefore, were to determine:

- If the Nd:YAG wavelength was suitable for nuclear ablation/emulsification.
- If available optical fibers could carry sufficient energy to bring about emulsification of the human cataract nucleus.

Fortunately, positive results were achieved, allowing the project to proceed.

Design of the actual probe occurred in an evolutionary manner with containment of laser energy a primary concern. A major advance was the ability to "lens" the end of the optical fiber to prevent beam divergence. A columnated beam provided a higher energy density for emulsification efficiency and permitted the beam to be confined within a metal-walled chamber. Anticipating that large pieces of the lens nucleus or even the edge of the whole nucleus would need to have access to the laser beam, a large opening to a "photovaporization chamber" was devised. To control aspiration flow, however, an aspiration tube with a 0.4-mm aspiration port was placed at the bottom of the photovaporization chamber. Large pieces of material could be drawn into the top of the photovaporization chamber to come in contact with the columnated laser beam. The resulting emulsified particles were aspirated from the bottom of the photovaporization chamber through the aspiration port into the aspiration tube. This probe design, having evolved over a 2-year period of experimentation, comprises the basis for the US patent awarded in 1987. The patent does not specify the wavelength of laser energy to be used nor does it limit the probe to intraocular use. It will, therefore, be possible to use the probe under patent protection with any laser energy source and configure the probe for use in any enclosed space in the body.

Safety and efficacy of the probe was examined in a variety of models. Initial tests were conducted using human cataract nuclei in vitro to confirm the effectiveness of the probe design on the target tissue (human cataracts). Safety testing proceeded in animal eyes, either enucleated or in vivo, with observation and histological verification of the absence of internal damage from stray laser energy. Having recently received FDA approval for initial clinical trials, it is anticipated that human testing will begin sometime during 1995.

Work is currently underway to determine the most effective surgical technique for cataract removal with the laser probe. At this time, surgery is being done through a scleral-tunnel incision and a small superiorly placed circular tear capsulotomy. Hydrodissection separates the lens nucleus from epinucleus and cortex. As the probe is inserted into the lens cortex, epinuclear material is aspirated and vaporized to allow room for the probe to lie adjacent to the nucleus. Photovaporization and aspiration of the nucleus proceeds from the equator inward. On occasion, use of a second instrument for manipulation of the nucleus has been necessary. The laser probe can be used for removal of the epinucleus and cortical material as well, but in some instances a standard irrigation/aspiration probe was necessary for total removal of the cortex. Since the amount of required movement of the probe inside the capsular bag usually is minimal, an endocapsular technique can often be used for lens removal.

The laser probe offers a number of potential benefits over the currently available ultrasonic devices:

Energy containment. Because of its patented design features (photovaporization chamber and a columnated laser beam), containment of energy is the hallmark of this device. Laser energy is confined within the metal tube of the probe tip (Figure 10-1). Breaking the posterior capsule requires a deliberate effort to engage the capsule and draw it into the laser path. The tissue action of the laser beam is limited to the confines of the photovaporization chamber, ie, there are no "distant effects" of the laser beam. The ultrasonic needle, however, can create vibrations in the fluid medium of the anterior chamber, setting up shock waves that may damage structures not touched directly by the needle itself.

Ease of use. Because the laser probe is similar in design to irrigation/aspiration handpieces already in use, the device can be considered user-friendly to most surgeons.

Reliability. The laser probe has no moving parts, and, therefore, has little opportunity to break during use. The two sub-parts most liable to usage wear (the aspiration tube and the laser delivery fiber) are projected to be single-use, disposable components.

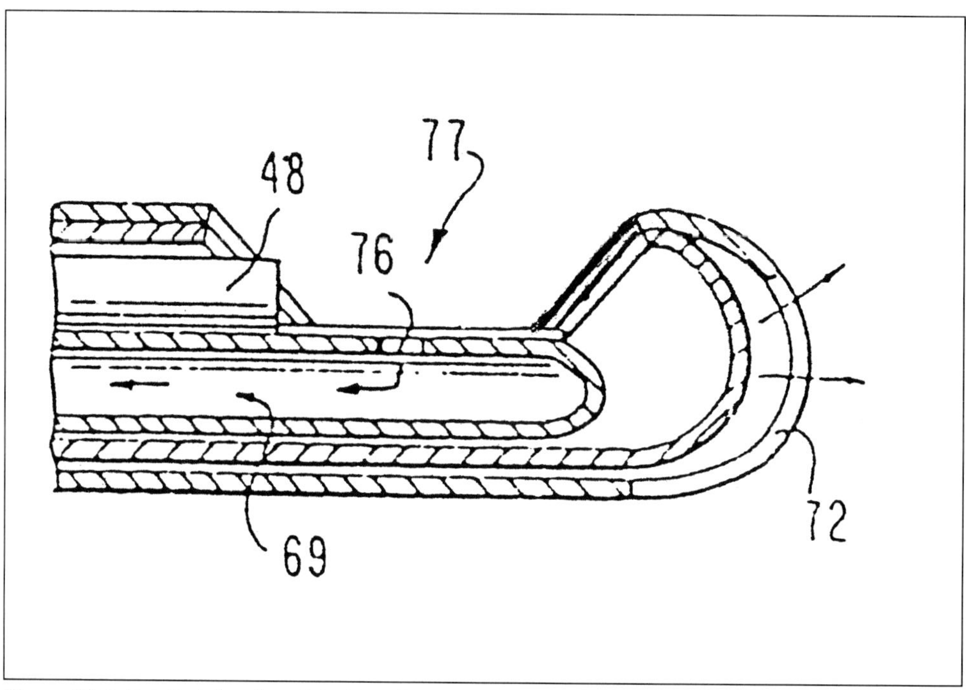

Figure 10-1. Detailed drawing of the Paradigm LaserPhaco Probe Tip. Key: 48=optical fiber/laser delivery, 69=aspiration tube, 72=irrigation tube, 76=aspiration port, 77=photovaporization chamber.

Versatility. As uses for the probe in other surgical specialties are developed, a single console can serve multiple surgeons, thus limiting a hospital's capital and financial exposure. Probes are currently under development that contain illumination and viewing capabilities to adapt to the requirements of non-ophthalmic surgical procedures.

The Paradigm System has an enormous potential to impact the manner in which surgery is performed in closed spaces of the human body, including the eye. The initial human surgical trial, cataract removal, will begin shortly to be followed by other applications as soon as possible. While no project in this stage of product development is guaranteed to come to a satisfactory conclusion, it is hoped that the theoretical and experimental foundation, successful so far, will lead to an effective and superior surgical device.

Chapter 11

Cataract Surgery Utilizing the Erbium Laser

D. Michael Colvard, MD
Richard P. Kratz, MD

Introduction

The Erbium laser, designed and manufactured by Premier Laser Systems in Irvine, California, is a multipurpose device for ophthalmic surgery. It is being developed for keratorefractive surgery, but has intraocular applications as well, which include continuous curvilinear capsulotomy, cataract extraction, glaucoma filtering procedures, and vitrectomy.

In this discussion, we will concentrate on the use of the Erbium laser in cataract surgery. We will review the general characteristics of the Erbium laser and describe laboratory work which has elucidated its tissue interactions during cataract extraction. Surgical techniques employed in Erbium laser cataract extraction will be discussed and several features of the device that we believe may ultimately offer advantages over ultrasonic technology for cataract extraction will be described.

General Characteristics of the Erbium Laser in Cataract Surgery

The Erbium laser has a number of qualities which make it well suited for intraocular use in cataract surgery. These include:

- Non-ultraviolet radiation
- Fiber optic delivery
- Capacity to ablate high water content tissue without a pigmented chromophore
- Ablation without thermal injury
- Smooth cutting capacity
- Cost-efficient manufacture, maintenance, and housing

Non-Ultraviolet Radiation

The Erbium laser produces infrared radiation with a wavelength of 2.94 microns, a wavelength which lies outside the range of ultraviolet radiation (Figure 11-1). For intraocular applications, this is very important as ultraviolet radiation is toxic to the corneal endothelium and to the retina and is potentially mutagenic.

Fiber Optic Delivery

Erbium energy can be delivered via a fiber optic system which can be coupled with an irrigation/aspiration device. This combination allows the surgeon to accomplish the entire procedure at a single sitting. Fiber optic delivery also allows for small incision size and use of small-incision intraocular lens technology (Figure 11-2).

Capable of Cutting Ocular Tissue

The Erbium laser wavelength is more highly absorbed in water than that of any other laser wavelength and therefore is ideal for cutting water-containing ocular structures such as the cataractous lens, sclera, vitreous, and cornea. Also, the high absorption of the 2.94 micron wavelength prevents the unwanted transmission and scatter of laser energy to adjacent and underlying tissues (Figure 11-3).

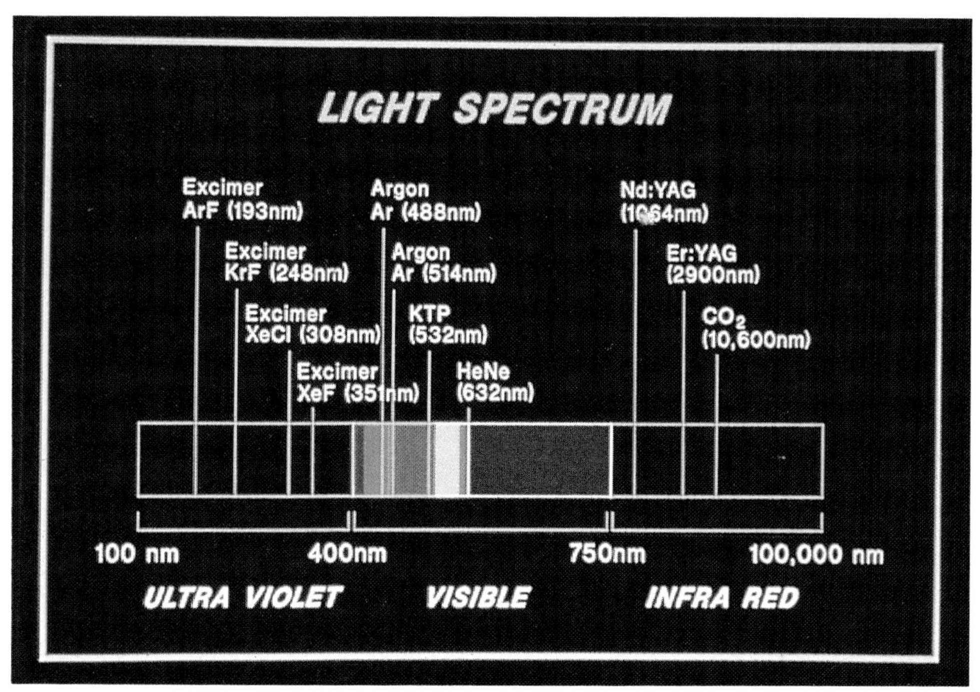

Figure 11-1. The Erbium laser produces infrared radiation.

Capable of Ablating Without Thermal Injury

Every laser has a thermal component, but the Erbium laser with maximal absorption in water has precise confinement of the laser energy deposition. The absorption of Erbium laser is approximately 1000 times greater than that of the Nd:YAG laser, 100 times greater than that of the Holmium laser, and 20 times greater than that of the CO_2 laser. Clearly, it is important to reduce the possibility of thermal damage and/or charring of ocular tissues with any ocular procedure.

For glaucoma procedures, non-thermal cutting may be particularly advantageous. By reducing thermal and mechanical energy to scleral, conjunctival, and episcleral tissues, it is believed that inflammation and scarring may be reduced. This may allow filtration procedures to be more predictable, titratable, and reliable (Figures 11-4A through 11-4C).

For cataract extraction, a reduction of the potential for thermal scatter is crucial for the protection of the corneal endothelium, the iris and ciliary body, and the capsule and the vitreous body.

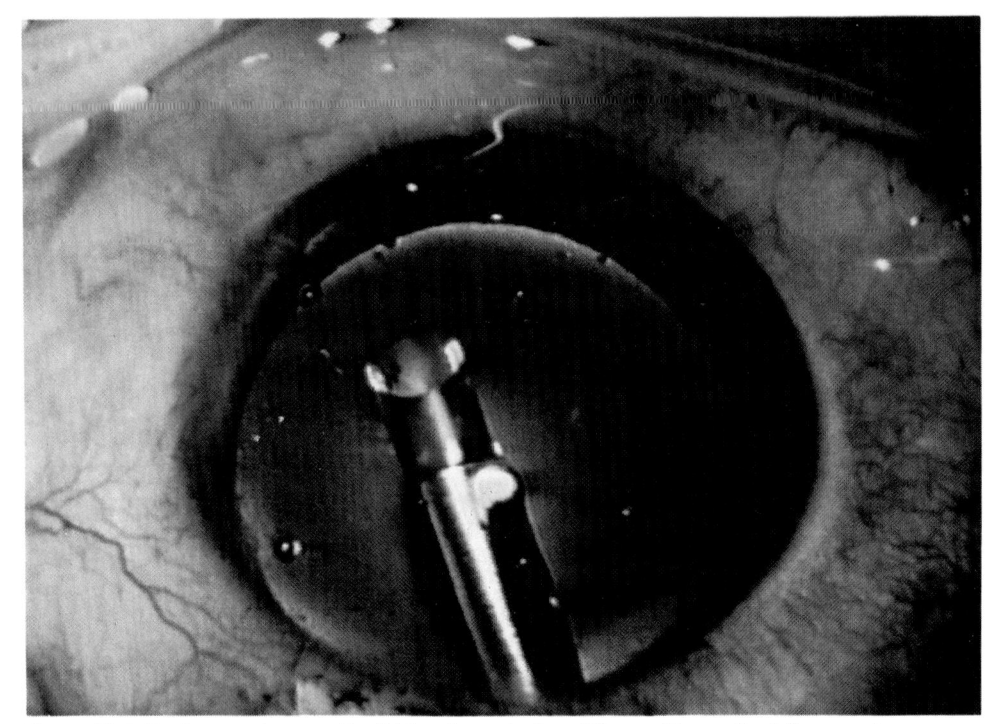

Figure 11-2. For intraocular use, the Erbium laser device utilizes a fiber optic delivery system.

Smooth, Non-Percussive Cutting

A circular anterior capsulotomy with a smooth, non-serrated capsular margin results in more reliable intraocular lens centration. Many surgeons find the manual continuous tear capsulotomy to be technically difficult to perform. The Erbium intraocular laser enables the surgeon to create a circular anterior capsulotomy by simply inscribing a circle on the surface of the anterior capsule with the same instrument that he or she would then use to remove the cataract. Although the Premier Erbium laser is not a continuous wave laser, it has been designed such that controlled movement of the laser probe at relatively high repetition rates with photoablative energy levels results in a capsular margin which is acceptably elastic (Figures 11-5A and 11-5B).

Cost-Efficient

The Erbium laser is a solid-state laser which produces its energy by exciting a crystal. Like its close relative, the neodymium-YAG laser, the Erbium YAG laser uti-

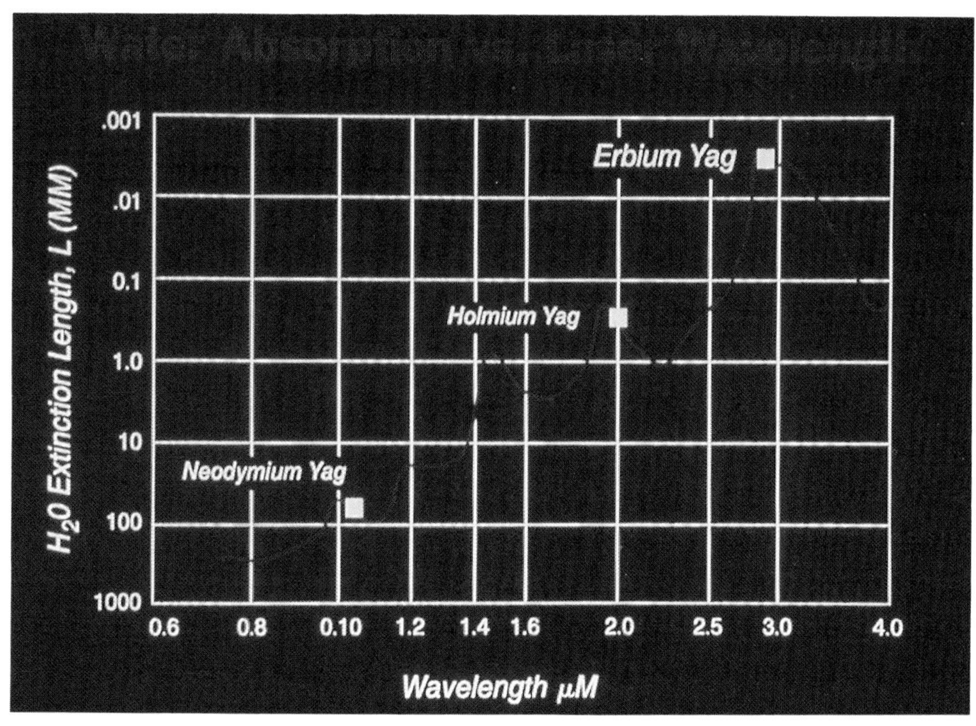

Figure 11-3. Erbium laser energy at 2.94 microns has the highest absorption in water of any known laser. This wavelength is ideal for the ablation of high water content structures such as cataract tissue, sclera, vitreous, and cornea.

lizes a yttrium-aluminum-garnet host crystal. The dopant or element which is placed within the crystal, however, is Erbium rather than neodymium. In terms of cost of manufacturing, durability, and reliability, the Erbium laser is similar to its better known neodymium cousin.

Unlike several other proposed "laser systems," the Erbium laser is approximately the size of a suitcase. It does not require a dedicated space. It can be moved easily and stored in a closet (Figure 11-6). There are no gases to replace and no specially trained engineers are needed. The laser is air cooled and can be plugged into a standard wall electrical socket.

By utilizing a fiber optic delivery system, the Erbium device is able to employ the most reliable and sophisticated tracking system in existence—the human surgeon. Expensive computerized tracking systems, which would increase the cost of each unit substantially, are unnecessary. Furthermore, because of the fiber optic delivery, the entire procedure with intraocular lens implantation can be performed in a single sitting at the operating table. Patients do not have to be treated twice and moved to two locations. Obviating the need for two separate procedures reduces the

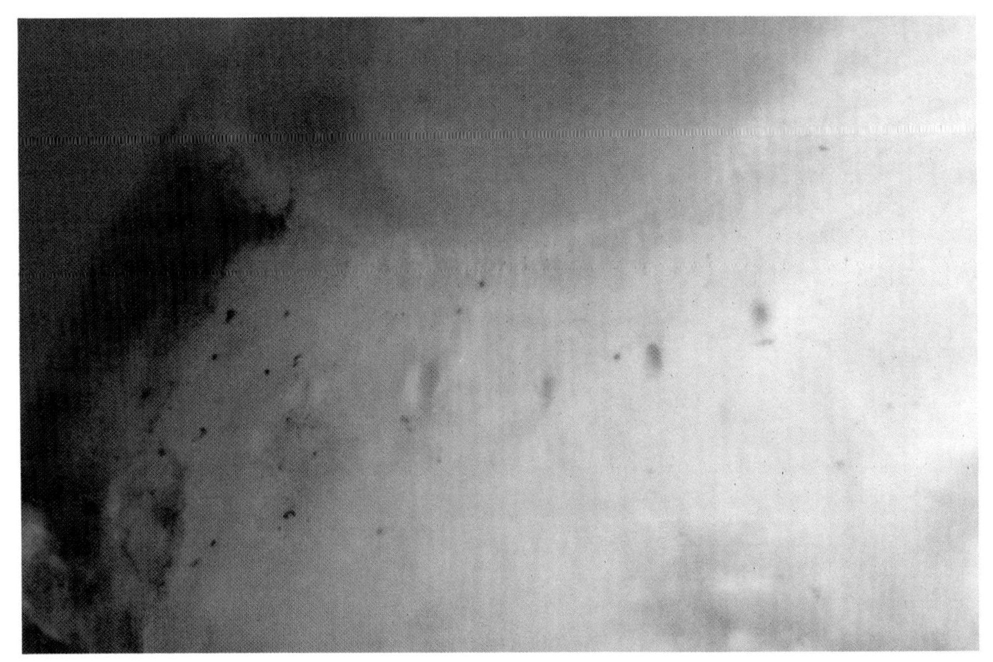

Figure 11-4A. Because of the high absorption of Erbium laser energy, there is less transmission of unwanted energy to adjacent and underlying areas. This precise containment of the laser energy results in less thermal damage to surrounding tissues than is seen with the Holmium or Nd:YAG lasers. This photograph demonstrates precise 320 micron sclerotomies in an eye bank eye.

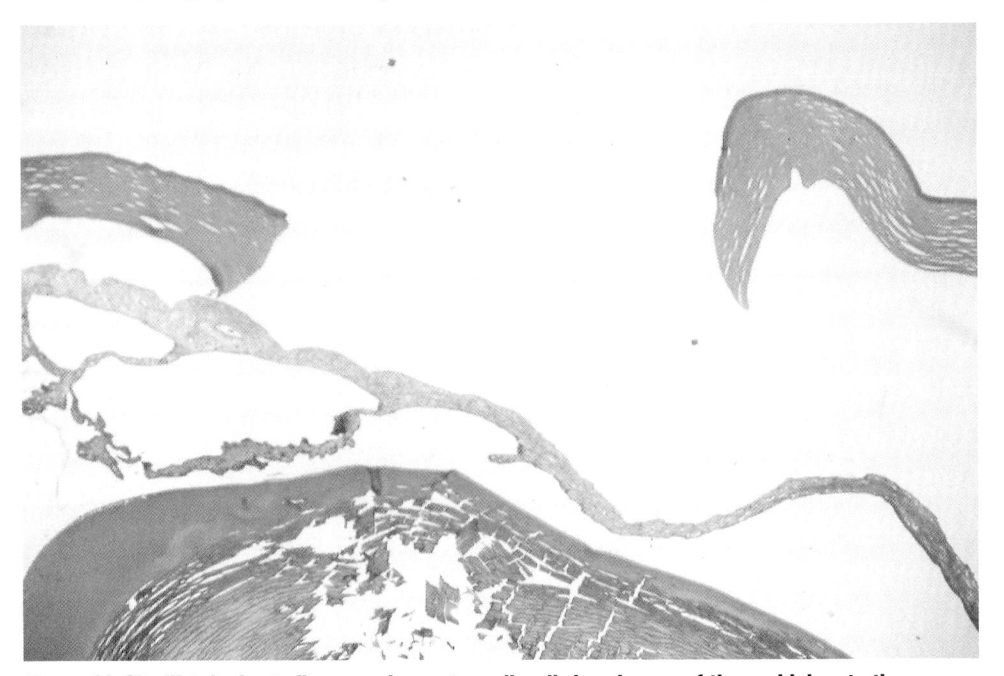

Figure 11-4B. Histologic studies reveal an extraordinarily low degree of thermal injury to tissues surrounding the sclerotomy sites.

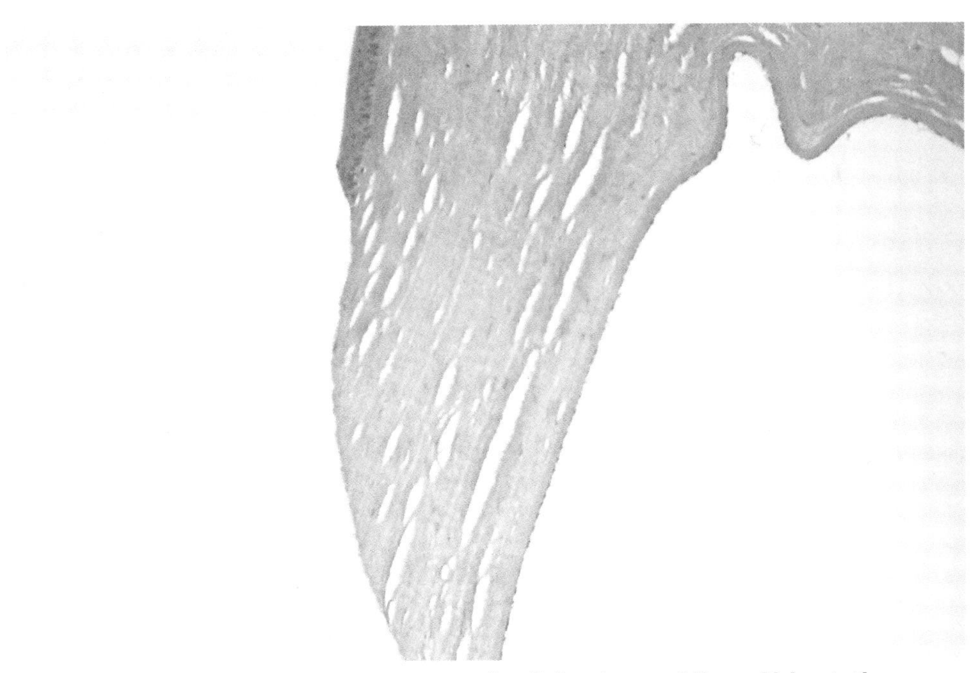

Figure 11-4C. Histologic studies reveal an extraordinarily low degree of thermal injury to tissues surrounding the sclerotomy sites.

operating cost for each procedure by reducing space and personnel needs, and by reducing the time needed by a surgeon to complete a procedure.

The development of a fiber, which could carry the Erbium wavelength reliably and cheaply, is one of the great technological challenges in the development of the Erbium laser intraocular device. While significant progress still must be made, the cost of semi-reusable fibers is predicted by Premier Laser Systems to be reasonably priced, and the per case cost of a cataract procedure is projected to be roughly equivalent to that of an "upscale" phacoemulsification procedure.

Erbium Laser Tissue Interactions During Cataract Extraction

The Erbium (Er: YAG) laser is a versatile laser which can be employed for procedures involving ocular tissues of any density. The pulsed Erbium laser energy interacts with tissue utilizing a combination of photoablative and photoacoustic phenomena.[1] The choice of one process over the other is dependent upon the surgi-

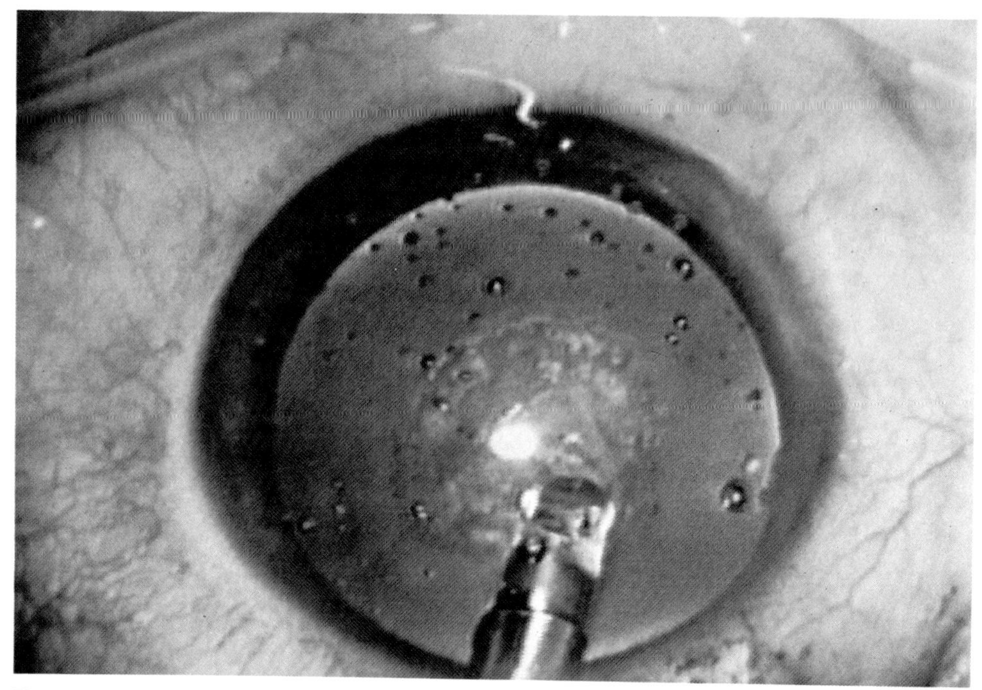

Figure 11-5A. The Erbium laser enables the surgeon to create a circular anterior capsulotomy by simply inscribing a circle on the surface of the anterior capsule.

cal procedure for which the Erbium laser is being utilized and can be controlled by appropriately adjusting the Erbium operating parameters of energy, repetition rate, pulse duration, and energy density.

When the device is used for anterior capsulotomy, photoablative properties are primarily employed. For this procedure the laser operating parameters are adjusted so that the delivered energy is just above the ablation threshold. This produces an incision in the capsular tissue with a clean margin. If the energy levels are delivered below the ablation threshold, a localized thermal reaction may be seen on the capsule and subcapsular surface. If energy levels are delivered which are significantly above that needed for ablation, one begins to witness photoacoustic effects. Photoacoustic effects result in a less regular capsular margin.

When emulsification of the cataractous lens is desired, the photoacoustic properties of the Erbium laser radiation are utilized. In this mode of operation, the Erbium laser behaves in a fashion substantially similar to an ultrasonic phacoemulsification device. Ultrasonic phacoemulsifiers operate primarily with acoustic energy generated by the cavitation created in a liquid environment. At the end of the

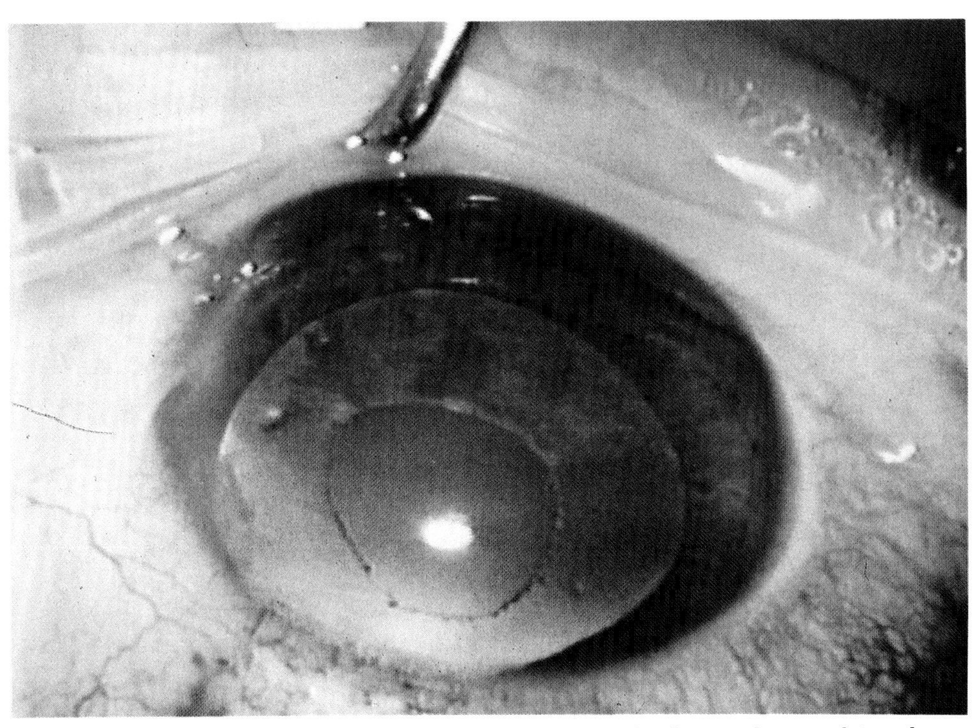

Figure 11-5B. The Erbium laser enables the surgeon to create a circular anterior capsulotomy by simply inscribing a circle on the surface of the anterior capsule.

ultrasonic probe's forward stroke, the tip impacts the lens. When the tip rapidly reverses direction, the fluid is unable to follow and a void is created in the liquid at the surface of the tip. When this void collapses, cavitation results which, in turn, produces a strong shock wave in the liquid. This shock wave propagates to the lens surface and mechanically disrupts the lens tissue.[2]

In a similar fashion, pulsed acoustic waves are created by the Erbium:YAG laser. This has been substantiated at Cedars Sinai Hospital in Los Angeles, California, where a group of researchers experimentally measured a strong photoacoustic component of the pulsed Erbium laser tissue interaction comparable to that of an acoustic phacoemulsification device.[3-6] The acoustic wave generated by the Er:YAG can be characterized by its impulse-induced pressure and by a pressure generated as a consequence of laser-induced cavitation in fluid. The impulse-induced pressure is generated when the laser pulse strikes the target tissue and removes a certain volume of the material. The cavitation-induced pressure is a result of the collapse of an Erbium laser pulse-induced bubble (Figures 11-7A through 11-7D).

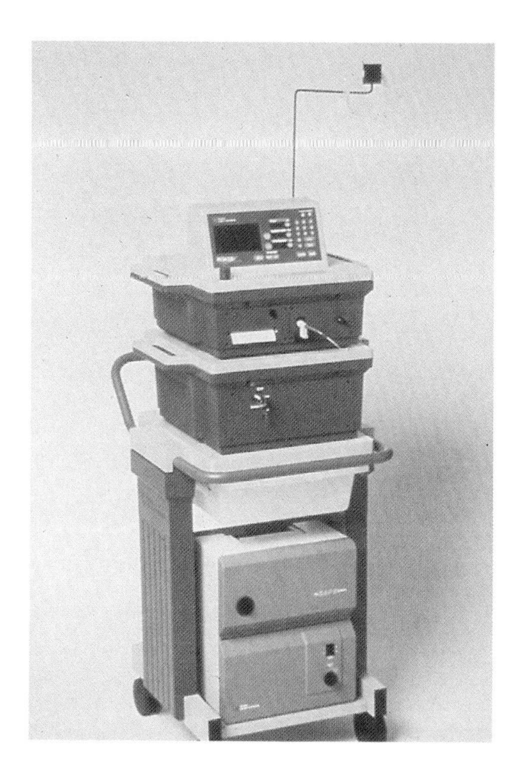

Figure 11-6. The solid-state Erbium laser is small, versatile, and similar in cost, durability, and reliability to the neodymium YAG laser.

Surgical Technique for Erbium Laser Cataract Extraction

The approach to cataract extraction using the Erbium laser fiber optic delivery system is similar to cataract extraction utilizing conventional ultrasonic techniques. The procedure is begun by reflecting the conjunctiva at the limbus. A scleral groove is made wide enough to allow the passage of the preferred intraocular lens. The incision is then dissected anteriorly and, if the surgeon desires, may be carried into clear cornea to produce a self-sealing internal corneal flap. A side-port incision may then be made at the limbus. This small incision generally measures approximately 1 mm in width and is self-sealing. The surgeon then places viscoelastic material in the anterior chamber to deepen the chamber and an entry is made into the anterior chamber under the scleral flap.

Anterior Capsulotomy

Anterior capsulotomy is then carried out. If viscoelastic material is used to deepen the anterior chamber, no irrigation is used with the laser fiber optic device. The device is introduced into the anterior chamber and the anterior capsulotomy is performed. If no viscoelastic material is used, the chamber may be maintained by utilizing the coaxial irrigation in the handpiece or by employing a side-port chamber maintainer. This deepens the anterior chamber and allows the anterior capsulotomy to be performed with simultaneous irrigation.

The anterior capsulotomy device consists of the Erbium fiber optic delivery system with a clear silica tip modified for this procedure. The tip used for anterior capsulotomy is a cylinder which has been polished so that there is a 45° wedge-shaped modification at the distal end of the probe. This 45° angle allows for the internal reflection of the laser energy. Laser energy which travels along the longitudinal axis of the fiber is thereby redirected at a 90° angle at the distal end of the laser tip. This tip modification focuses the laser energy directly toward the anterior capsule (Figure 11-8).

The capsulotomy probe allows the surgeon to see the capsule through the clear tip and allows the surgeon to visualize the lasing action of the Erbium device during the process of anterior capsulotomy. There are no opaque structures that interfere with visualization, and the surgeon is able to carefully monitor and modify the capsulotomy design as he or she proceeds.

The capsulotomy is carried out by inscribing a circular pattern on the surface of the anterior capsule. Although it is possible to visualize the capsule easily during the lasing procedure when the pupil is wide, it is also possible to lase under the iris. This is particularly useful when the pupillary dilation is poor (Figures 11-9A and 11-9B).

The laser spot size with this device is approximately 800 microns. For anterior capsulotomies, it has been found that a repetition rate of 10 Hz with an energy setting of 12 to 15 mJ gives the best results. At these prescribed parameters, the capsulotomy is smooth with evidence of a pseudomembranous reaction on the surface of the capsule. Since the laser is not a continuous wave laser, it is necessary to move in a relatively slow and controlled fashion, as one draws the circle. If a complete circle is not completed on the first pass for whatever reason, it is possible to go back and restart or "touch up" certain areas of the circular opening. Starting and restarting the laser does not result in a capsular margin defect if one takes care to connect the edges of the unfinished capsulotomy.

Cataract Extraction

Following the completion of the anterior capsulotomy, hydrodissection and hydrodelineation is accomplished. Hydrodissection consists of injected BSS under the anterior capsulotomy, separating the nucleus and cortical material from the capsular

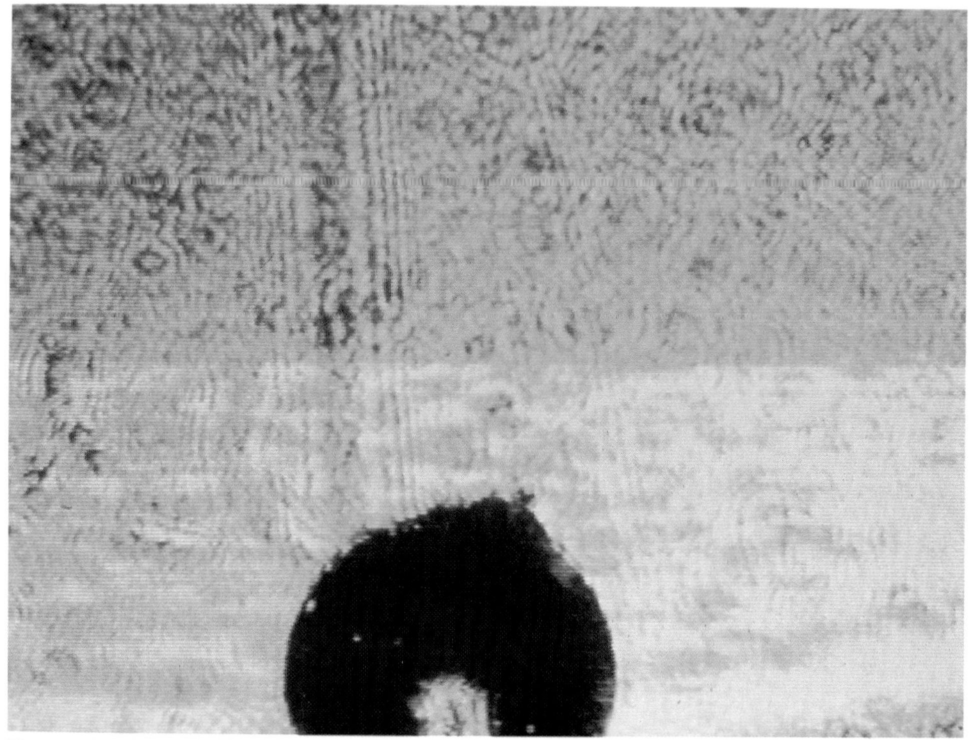

Figure 11-7A.

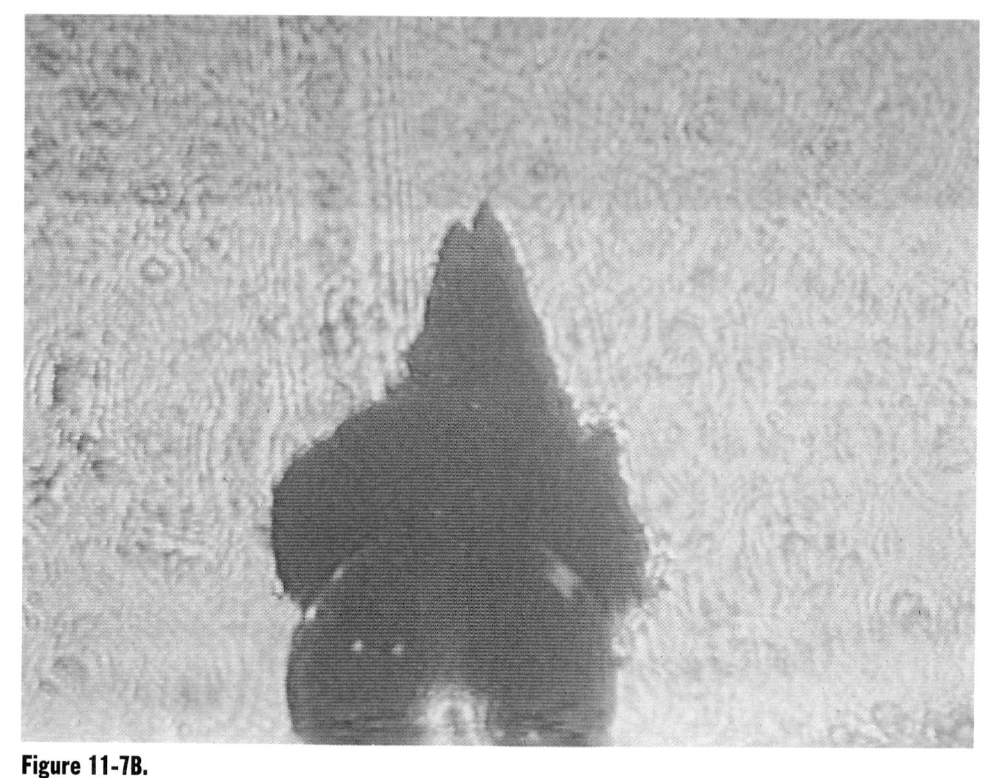

Figure 11-7B.

The Erbium laser creates a cone-shaped cavitation bubble at the end of the probe. Implosion of this bubble generates an acoustic wave capable of emulsifying cataract tissue. Figures 11-7A through 11-7D demonstrate the generation and collapse of this bubble.

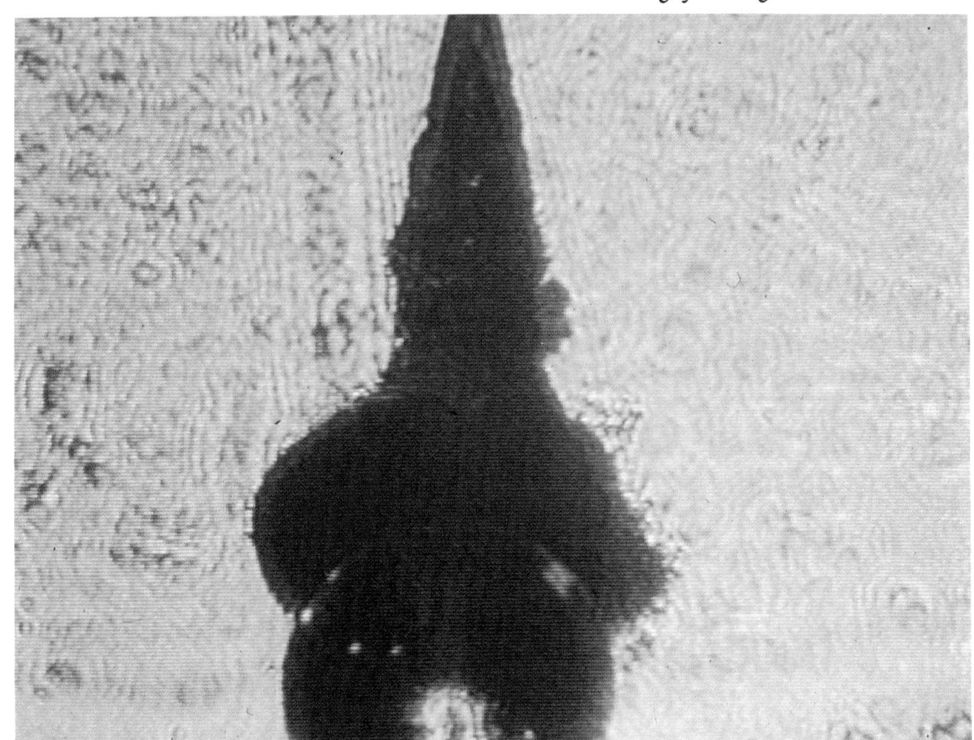

Figure 11-7C.

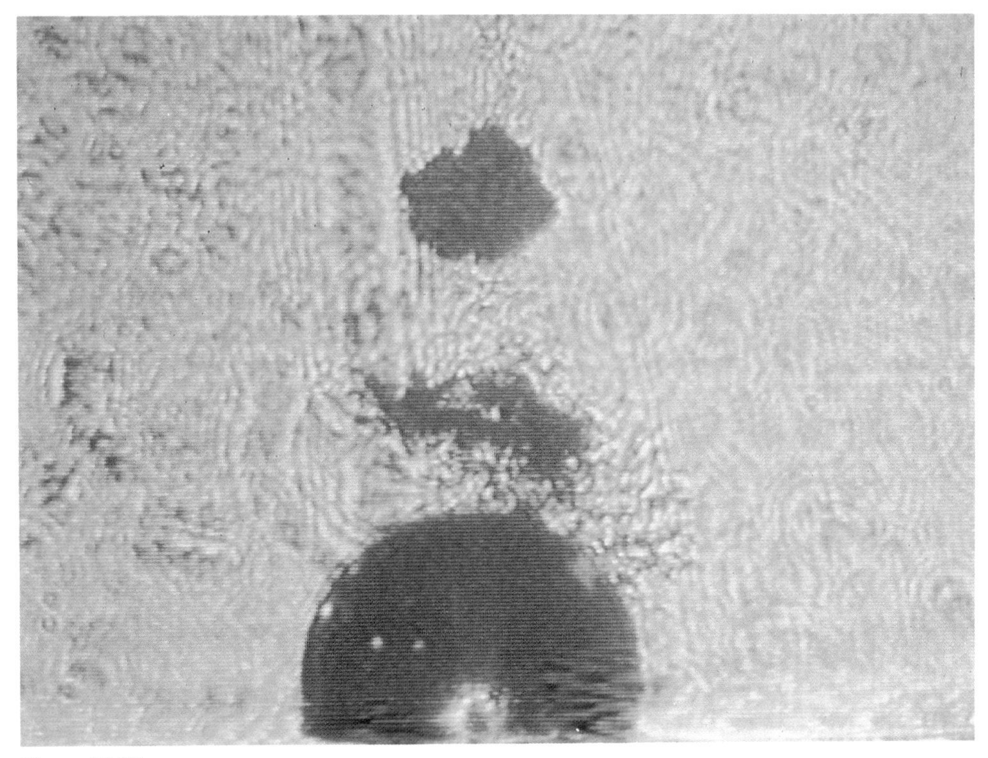

Figure 11-7D.

bag. Hydrodelineation consists of separating the nucleus from the cortex and the epinuclear material with BSS. The Erbium laser cataract device is then introduced into the anterior chamber. A lens emulsification tip is employed, rather than a capsulotomy tip. The lens emulsification tip consists of a silica probe which has a smooth spherical distal end. With this probe, the laser energy travels along the longitudinal axis of the fiber and continues through the probe tip along this longitudinal axis.

Several different aspiration irrigation systems have been used with the Erbium laser. The most basic approach utilizes a chamber maintainer for irrigation and a cannula-like aspiration device brought through a side-port. The laser fiber is then introduced at the site of the primary incision. This technique was utilized in the initial clinical series performed by one of the authors (DMC) (Figures 11-10A through 11-10D). Alternatively aspiration, irrigation, or both may be introduced coaxial to the laser fiber.

Lens extraction is accomplished by simply painting the surface of the cortical and nuclear materials centrally with the laser probe. The activation of the lasing process results in a gradual flaking of the nuclear material. These small flakes of nuclear material are then aspirated. As one lases the nuclear material, one has the sensation of erasing the cataractous tissue.

The laser lens emulsification tips produce spot sizes between 400 and 800 microns. The repetition rate is generally set between 10 and 15 Hz and energy levels are set between 20 and 60 mJ. Higher energies are only used for the very dense central nuclear material. As one approaches softer cortical material, the energy levels are reduced significantly to afford a less energetic lasing action.

In our initial clinical series we elected to lase only the anterior and central nuclear material. Further clinical experience is needed to determine the optimal levels of energy when lasing is performed close to the posterior capsule.

After the nuclear material has been lased, the aspiration system is used to remove the epinuclear and cortical material. Epinuclear material may be lased at low energy levels to facilitate its aspiration. The laser device is then withdrawn from the anterior chamber, the posterior capsule is polished, and the intraocular lens is introduced.

Potential Advantages of Erbium Laser in Cataract Surgery

The Erbium laser provides the surgeon with a very simple way to perform a smooth circular anterior capsulotomy. The continuous curvilinear capsulotomy has

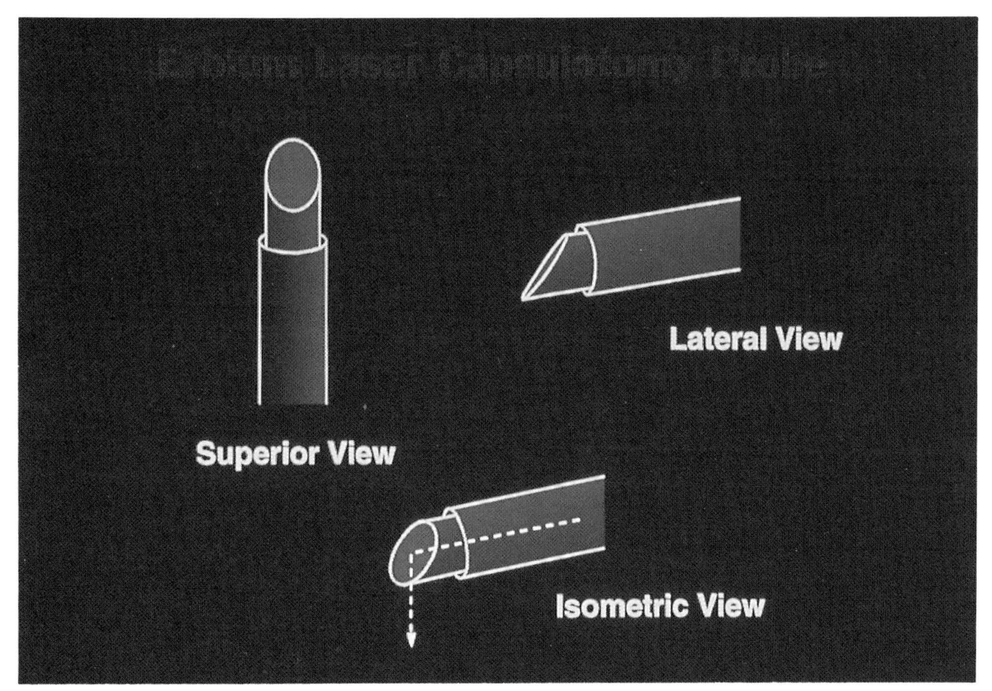

Figure 11-8. The anterior capsulotomy probe redirects laser energy at 90° to the axis of the fiber. This tip modification focuses the laser energy directly toward the anterior capsule.

several well-accepted advantages over more traditional "can opener" style capsulotomies. The technique for tearing a circular opening in the anterior capsule mechanically, however, can be challenging and is particularly difficult in patients with poorly dilating pupils. The Erbium laser device allows the surgeon to fashion a circular anterior capsulotomy by simply drawing a circle on the anterior capsule. The Erbium laser circular capsulotomy is resistant to the development of radial tears, and after lens implantation, carries all the postoperative advantages of a manual continuous tear capsulotomy. With further development the Erbium laser may offer several advantages over ultrasonic and mechanical methods for cataract extraction. The handpiece of the Erbium laser device utilizing a fiber optic delivery system is extraordinarily light and may be maneuvered by the surgeon in the anterior and posterior chamber with more ease and control than existing ultrasonic handpieces. The laser handpiece is approximately the size and the weight of a pencil; it is well balanced and comfortable to hold and manipulate. Unlike ultrasonic phacoemulsification devices, there are no heavy hoses running from the posterior aspect of the device. The fiber carrying the energy and the irrigation and aspirating tubes are collectively no heavier or bulkier than three thin silicone tubes.

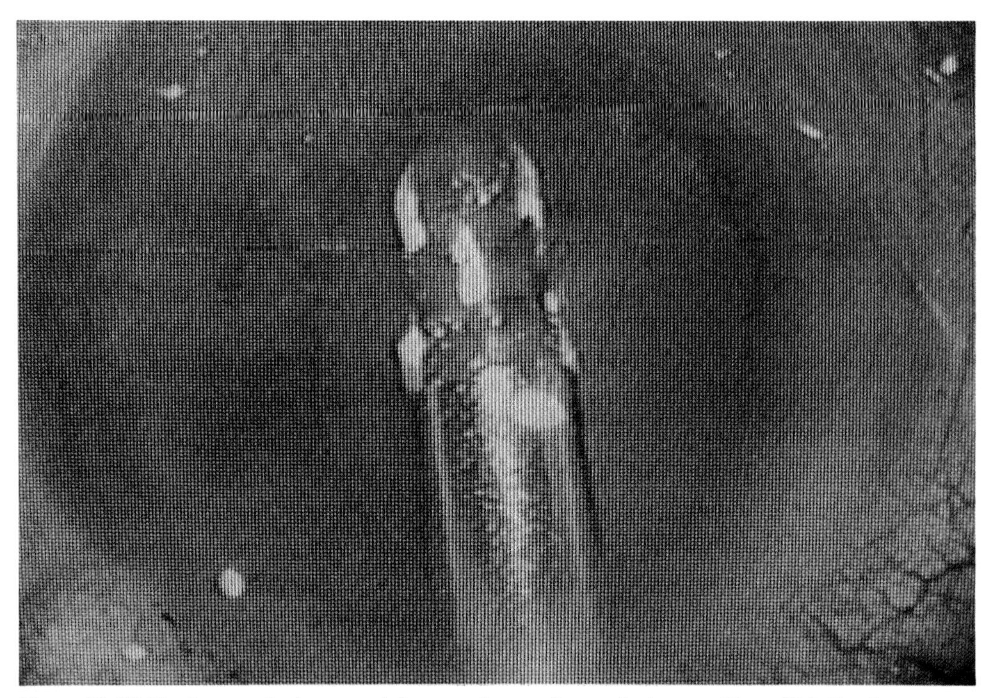

Figure 11-9A. The laser anterior capsulotomy probe can be used when pupillary dilatation is poor. The device allows circular capsulotomies to be performed in eyes on which mechanical capsulorhexis would be difficult to perform.

The tip of the laser fiber is smooth and spherical. There are no points or needle-like projections, and the emulsifying action of the Erbium laser during lens removal appears to be very gentle. When ablating and emulsifying cataract tissue with the Erbium laser, one has only to stroke the surface of the nuclear material with the smooth olive-tip probe. The cataract material is gradually reduced in size. The emulsified material, consisting of tiny flakes of the nucleus in suspension, is easily aspirated. One has the sensation of simply erasing the nuclear material. If techniques can be developed whereby energy levels are gradually lowered to reduce the lasing activity to a gentle agitation, the potential for greater protection of the posterior capsule may be possible.

Erbium laser technology may ultimately allow surgeons to perform cataract extraction entirely within the endocapsular envelope through a small opening. Such an endocapsular procedure will be desirable once an elastic injectable intraocular lens material has been developed and perfected and the problems of long-term capsular opacification are solved.

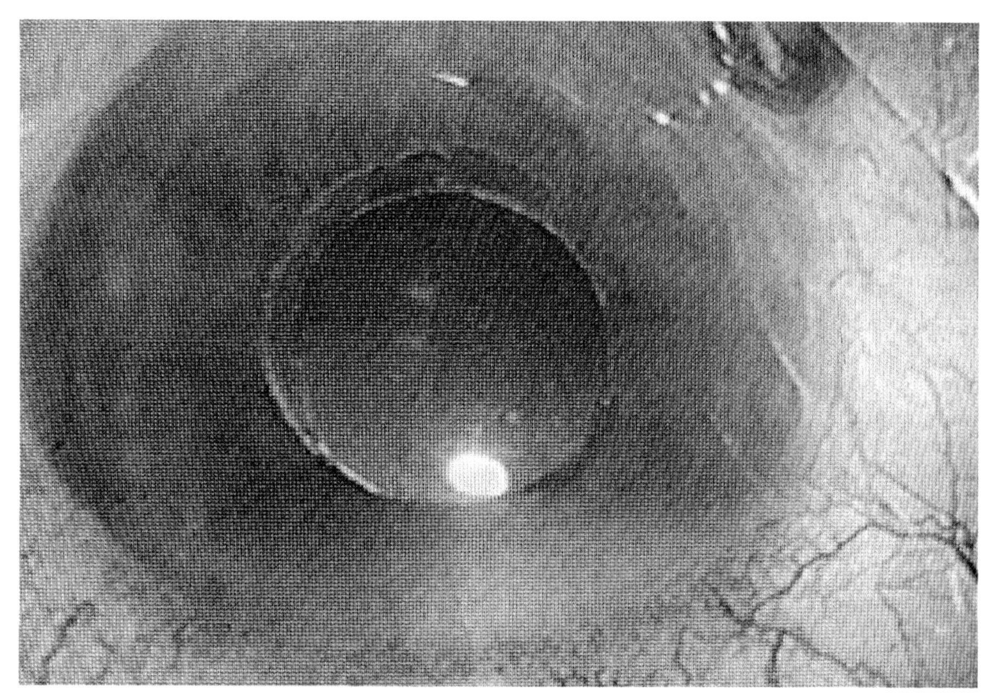

Figure 11-9B. The laser anterior capsulotomy probe can be used when pupillary dilatation is poor. The device allows circular capsulotomies to be performed in eyes on which mechanical capsulorhexis would be difficult to perform.

Summary

In this chapter, we have presented an overview of the Erbium laser in cataract surgery. We have discussed the characteristics of the Erbium wavelength and the physics of its tissue interactions as well as the surgical techniques presently being employed for cataract extraction. The device has potential advantages over existing ultrasonic technology for cataract extraction which include:

- Ability to perform circular capsulotomies.
- A handpiece with superior ergonomics.
- A smooth, spherical olive-tip probe without sharp edges or points.
- A potentially more gentle lens cutting mechanism.

It is possible that these features may help to make cataract surgery safer and that Erbium laser cataract extraction may have a shorter learning curve than is encoun-

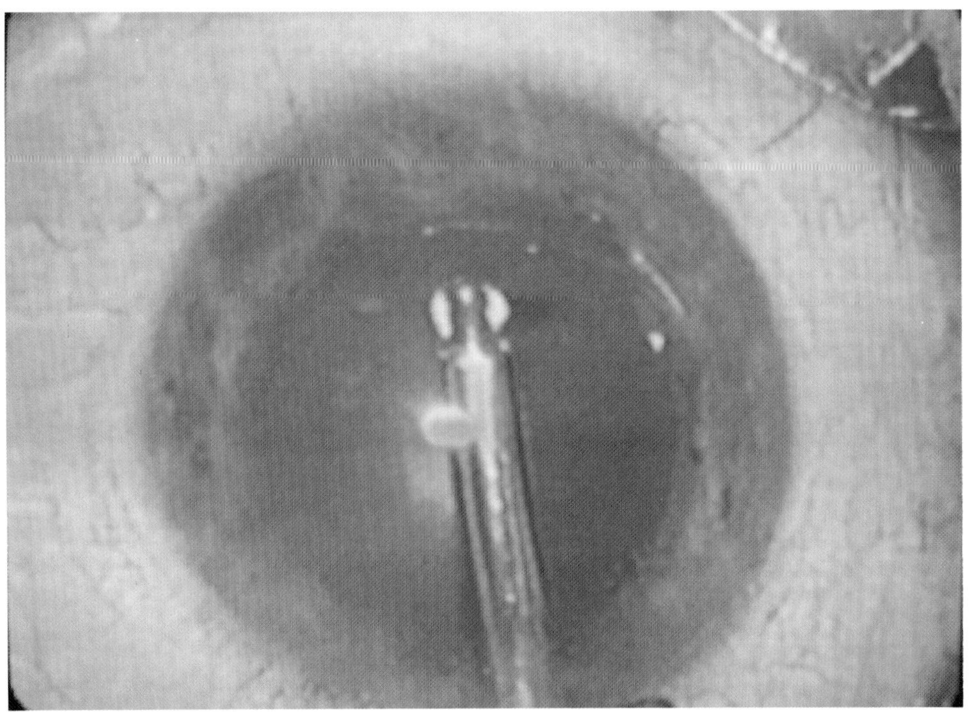

Figure 11-10A. In the initial clinical series, a circular capsulotomy was performed using the capsulotomy probe.

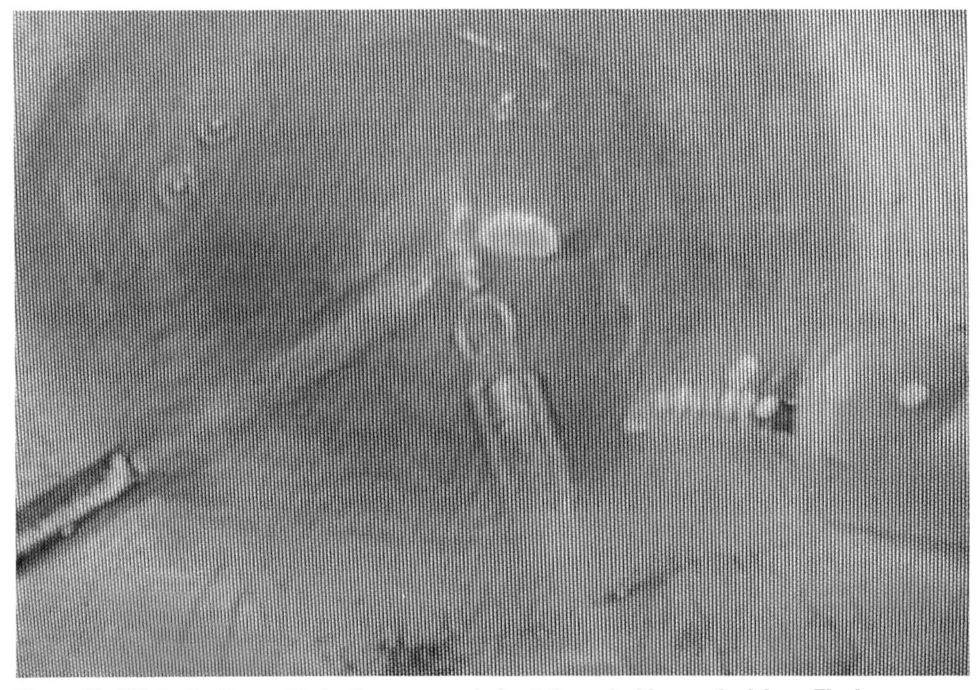

Figure 11-10B. Aspiration and irrigation was carried out through side-port incisions. The laser cataract extraction probe was introduced through the primary incision. The lasing action was used to bring the anterior and central nuclear material into suspension.

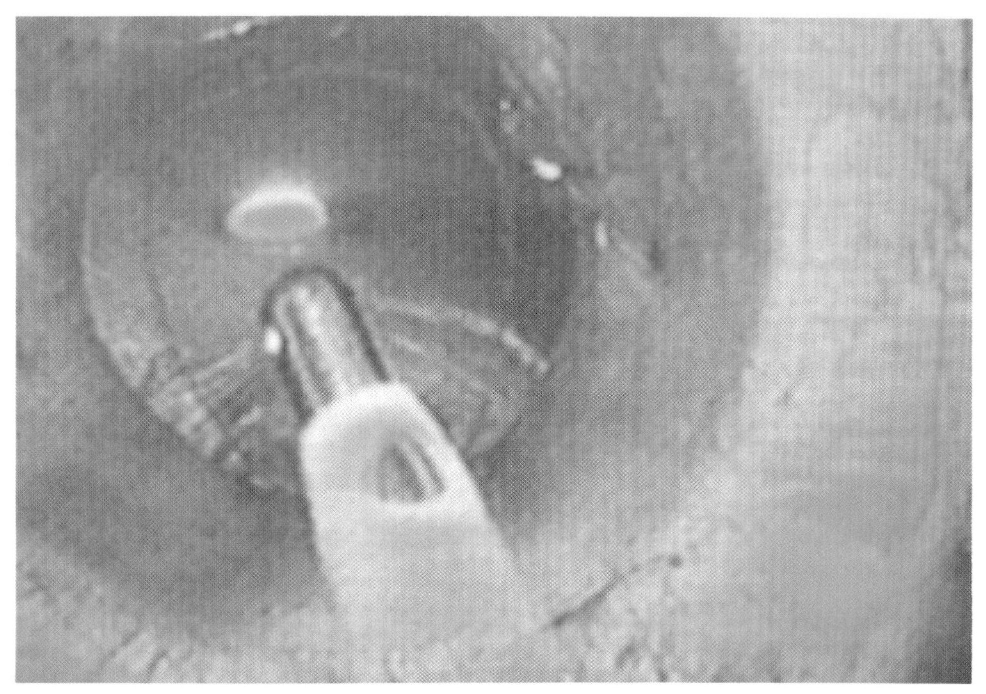

Figure 11-10C. The cortical material was aspirated in the customary fashion.

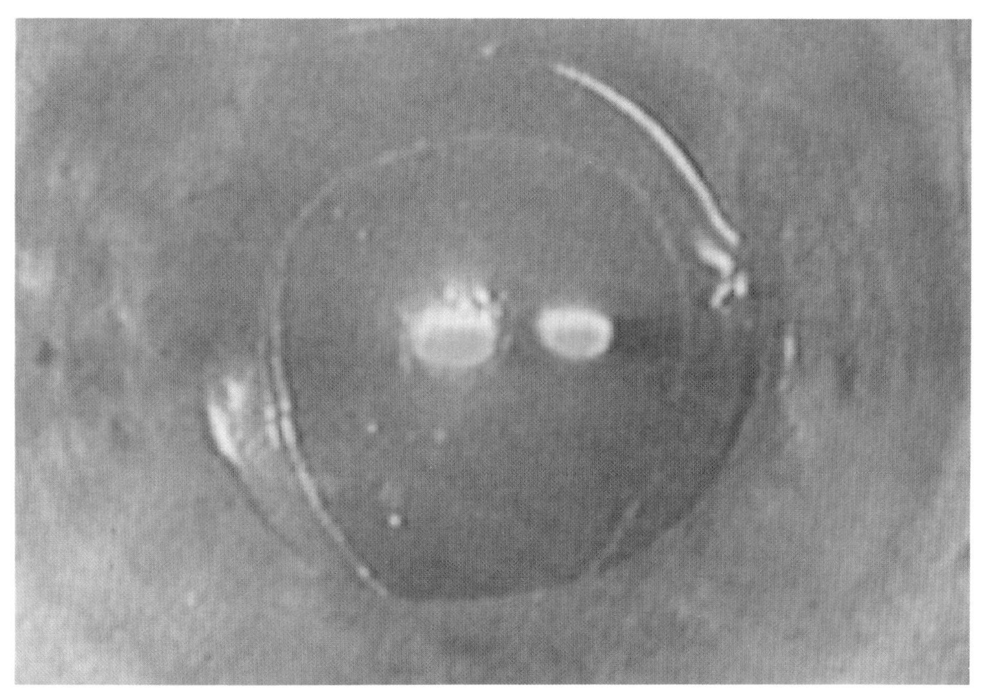

Figure 11-10D. A standard PMMA intraocular lens was implanted.

tered with ultrasonic phacoemulsification devices. If the potential of the Erbium laser becomes fully realized in cataract surgery, the device may help to make small-incision surgery more accessible for a greater number of surgeons and bring the advantages of small-incision surgery to a greater number of patients worldwide.

References

1. Boulnois JL. *Laser Is Medical Science*. Balliere Tindall; 1986.
2. SBIR grant Er:YAG Laser Lens Emulsification.
3. Loertscher H, Shi WQ, Grundfest WS. Tissue ablation through water with Er:YAG lasers. Accepted for publication in *IEEE Transaction on Biomedical Engineering*.
4. Shi WQ, Loertscher H, Vari SG, Grundfest WS. Tissue interaction with mid-infrared lasers in saline. *Bulletin Amer Phys Society*. 1991;36(7)1978.
5. Shi WQ, Steinmetz DA, Vari SG, Grundfest WS. Ho:YAG induced cavitation and the associated pressure wave generation. Submitted to CLEO 92. May 1992.
6. Shi WQ, Snyder WJ, Vari SG, Grundfest WS. Ho:YAG laser impulse induced pressure in soft tissues. Submitted to CLEO 92. May 1992.

Index